Dedication

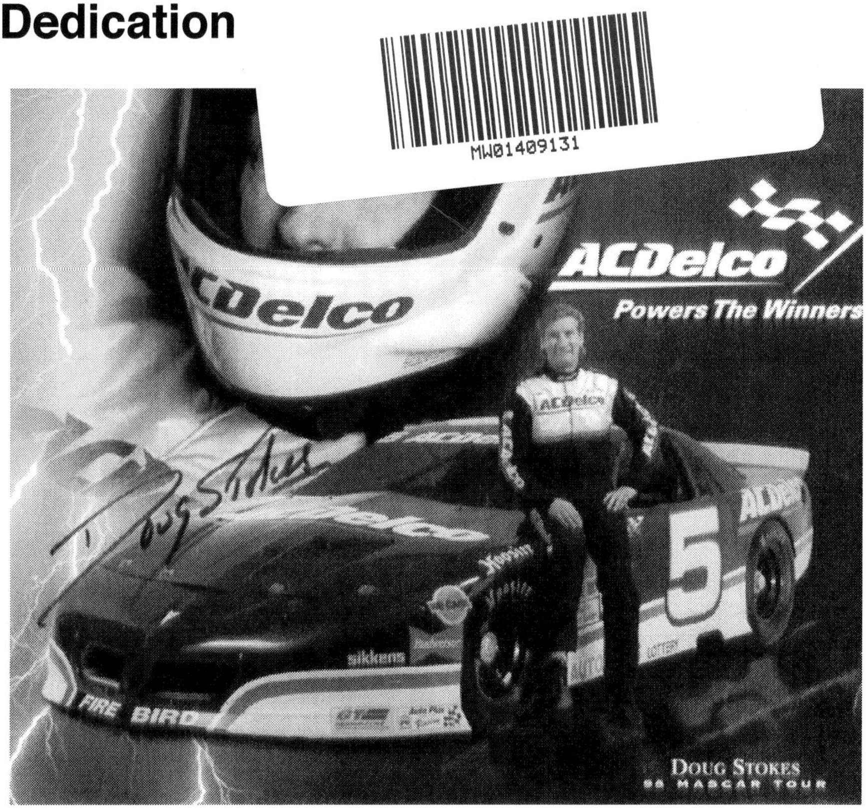

Doug Stokes, my father, has been my inspiration throughout my life. Doug was at the height of a multimillion dollar career when he left all his business enterprises to pursue his life long dream of becoming a professional stock car driver.

My father's support has been instrumental in my success. His energy and drive to pursue life to the fullest has motivated me to always be the very best that I can be for both myself and my patients.

I have been blessed to have Doug Stokes as my father. For all that he has given me, I most appreciate him teaching me not just to dream the impossible dream but to pursue it.

-Buckwheat

Acknowledgments

With joy and pleasure, I thank all my clients, teachers, family and friends who have totally supported me throughout my career and encouraged me to share my knowledge through the many years it has taken me to write this book.

I wish to first thank my wife Katherine, who has made all things possible in my life. You are the reason I consider every day a gift. You are my best friend and I love you. In a sense you are the reason I wrote this book because you kept telling me I would be able to write it, even when I doubted myself you always had faith in me.

My mother, Rosalind is also instrumental in who I am today. She was the perfect mother and provided an upbringing that can only be summarized as magical. When I was a young boy every-day was exciting, mainly because of the active role my mother took in raising her children. A great cook, caring parent and not bad poet, my mother was the philosophical doorway to the esoteric. I remember, even at an early age, long conversations around the fireplace concerning life after death, metaphysics and the realm of possibilities. Great memories I often revisit.

How can I not thank my sister Raylene. She was always the Yin to my Yang personality. Always taking up for me, even when I was at fault and really just being there for me as you would expect a great sister to be. I am inspired by her ability to maintain a successful law practice while being the perfect mom to her 3 beautiful children. She is deserving in every way.

There are many others who have had a role in shaping the physician I have become. Thank you, Dr. Joe Rogers, Dr. Michael Gillespie, Dr. Gary Goerg, Dr. Mike Fiscella, Dr. Robert Wootton, Dr. John Amano, Dr. Ted Carrick, Dr. Jeff Rockwell, Dr. Jeffery Bland, Dr. Karel Lewit, Dr. Alan Dyer, Paul Ellis, Dr. Brain Synder, Dr. Hans Jurgen, Dr. Phillip Greenman, Dr. John Sarno, Dr. Richard Preblish and Dr. David Seaman. I am humbled by your wisdom and dedication to the healing arts.

Forward

This book, Heal Yourself: The 7 Steps To Innate Healing, will present, in detail, a logistical road map to rediscovering your health. Regardless of the diagnosis, this approach works. Unlike many doctors who publish books, Dr. Stephen Stokes is a working physician who treats patients everyday. Frustrated with traditional allopathic treatments that just masking symptoms, Dr. Stokes developed an effective protocol to help patients overcome illness and pain without invasive procedures or dangerous drugs. In Dr. Stephen Stokes own words,

Disease is a systemic event and not isolated or compartmentalized as modern medicine claims. Everything is connected and you cannot treat one area of the body without affecting another. When I stopped treating the condition and focused on healing the patient, that is when I began to experience miracles in my clinic. Why? The answer is simple. I had tapping into the most powerful medicine available, the body's innate ability to heal itself. Innate is a term that has been shelved in today's drug driven culture but it is still the only way our body's get better. I listen to innate, offer my help and then get out of it's way. All true healing happens in this way.

Anyone looking for a more healthy life filled with energy and freedom from pain will find essential information within these pages. This book is a manual to uncover your optimal potential and join the thousands of people, just like you, that have overcome illness and reached their optimal potential. I would encourage all readers to study the information within these pages and if in the Southwest Florida area, make an appointment to see Dr. Stokes personally. I use these very same protocols on my own patients and family with unsurpassed success.

Dr. Michael P. Gillespie DC, B.Sc., BSE
Assistant Professor, Dept. of Health Professions
CUNY York College

Heal Yourself

The 7 Steps To Innate Healing

Dr. Stephen Stokes B.Sc., DC, FIAMA, CF(o)

2012

Crazy Fish Publishing
Cape Coral, Florida

Crazy Fish Publishing
Cape Coral, Florida 33914

First published by Crazy Fish Publishing 3/07/2012

ISBN: 978-1-105-58577-7

Printed in the United States of America

This book is printed on acid-free paper.

The views expressed in this work are solely those of the author and do not necessarily reflect the views of the publisher, and the publisher hereby disclaims any responsibility for them. The information contained herein is not intended to treat or diagnose any condition and is offered for educational purposes only. Always consult with a trained physician before undertaking any sort of self treatment. Many supplements and herbs can have dangerous side effects when combined with prescription medications. It is not recommended that persons currently taking prescription medications attempt to follow any information contained within this book without the approval of their primary care physician.

Testimonials

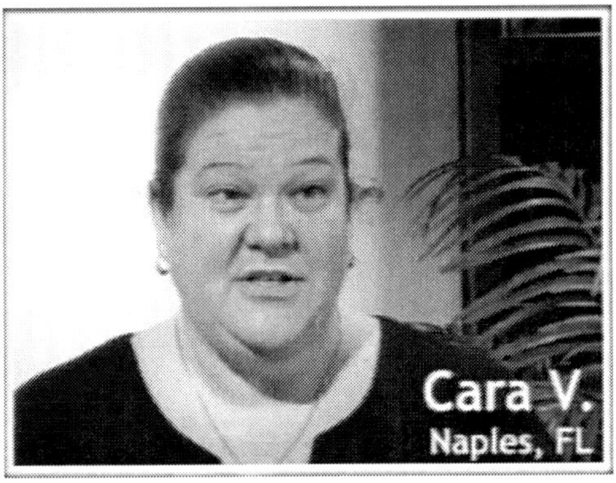

The pain that I was experiencing was crushing. It was hard and heavy and it felt like something was compressing my spine. Sleeping was a major problem for me and if you don't sleep you end up miserable. Dr. Stokes gave me the breath that I hadn't taken in years. I mean you just stand around gritting your teeth and being horribly in pain and then all of a sudden you get relief and it's like aaaaah! At the 11th treatment I was a little better, by the 20th treatment I was like wow... it was better. You should try everything you can to correct things without going to extreme measures. I have to say that this was not the place that I started but inevitably it was the place that healed my wounds. Dr. Stokes is very friendly, down-to-earth, the medical assistants are very sweet, they know what they're doing. It puts you at ease when somebody can answer all your questions without hesitation that's a bonus to me in any kind of work.

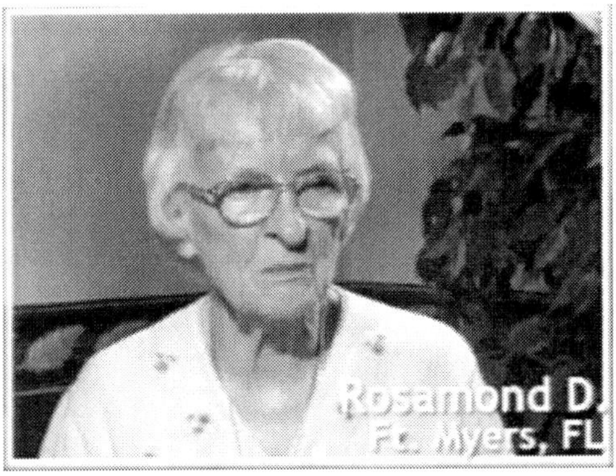

I don't even know how to explain the pain. It was really bad and I could hardly walk. Now after treatment, I can get out of bed without pain and that's a biggie for me. It stretches the disc and helps bring the fluid back in and that's what it did. Come to Dr. Stokes, he's one in a million and his treatment is a real help to humankind.

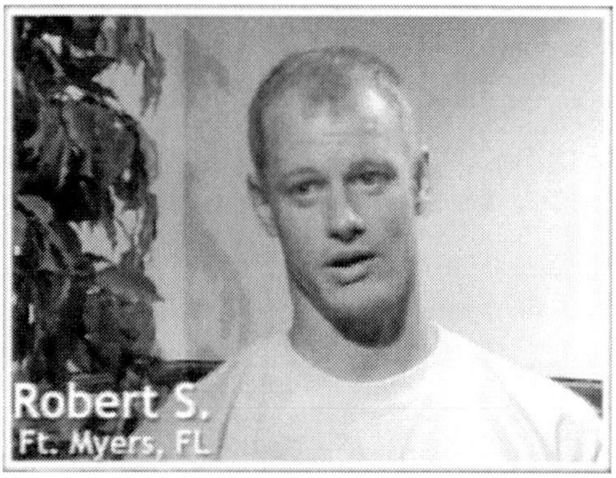

Couldn't sit or lay down, couldn't stand, couldn't bend, could not do anything. I was in constant pain. Now I am lifting more than I was before the injury. I had these pains, tweaks and aches. I thought it was just the work I do. Turns out I had underlying problems going back years. After the first treatment and cheating by being on pain medicine I thought I was cured and started jumping up and down acting crazy, just happy that I had less pain. They calmed me down and explain what was going on. They had to ween me off the painkillers and continue treating, then after two weeks I was feeling really good, was walking normally, was lifting, I could bend over and I was sleeping at night. I was noticing changes. I had met a couple of people that had surgery and they had lost function. They were never the same. I need to be mobile, surgery was not an option for me. I love the staff, they work with you. I never had insurance coverage, I had a little bit of money in the bank but not much. I let the doctor know up front I probably couldn't afford the treatments. They worked with me, they said don't worry about that, we are going to get you better and they did.

I guess I could say I had severe pain a minimum of 10 years. Well, it sure is better and it's amazing, it forms a suction I guess and it sucks the disc back in. It's amazing. I don't know anything else that can do that. Dr. Stokes treatments have helped me a lot.

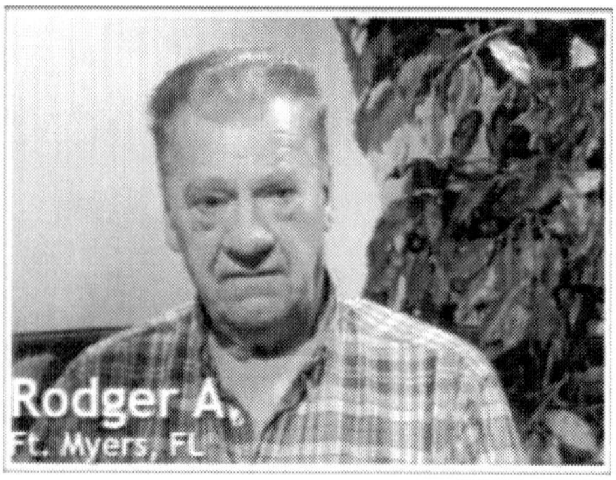

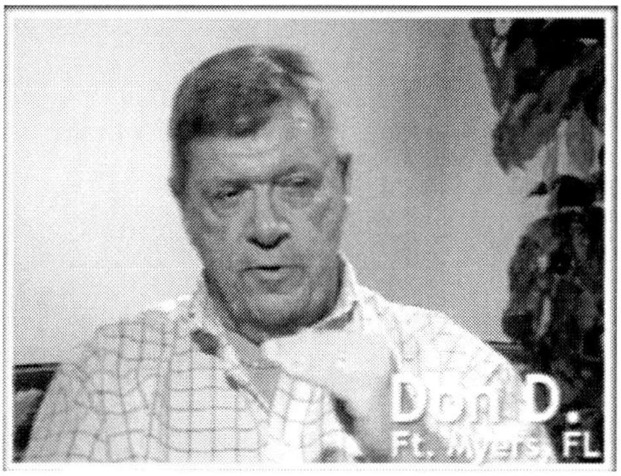

I had a very hard time straightening up in the morning, had to stand in a hot shower to get the pain to subside a little bit. Now I feel like a new person. I went from 60 down to 40. I am kidding, I am not really 60 but I really, truly think this is the greatest thing that ever happened because I didn't need surgery or anything. My office noticed a big difference in how I walk. I was walking without a limp, I wasn't bent over, you know, just tremendous change. I have an ex-wife in Pittsburgh who had back surgery, she's never been the same. This was my very last option and it worked, nobody cut me or anything. Definitely come in and see Dr. Stokes and he'll talk with you, do an exam and tell you what the problem is. I would just come in and relaxed on the table and after I felt like a new person.

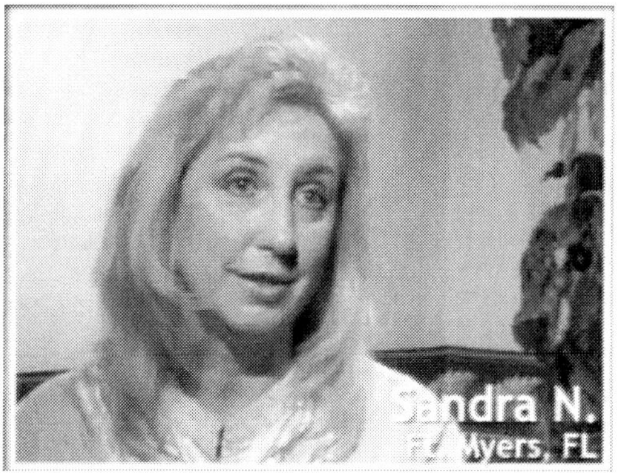

I was in tremendous amount of pain, my hobby is horse back riding and I just had no interest in it whatsoever. Well, I'm back horseback riding! I have a 10 year-old and I enjoy activities with him. Before it would hurt to do anything. So it's really made a huge difference in my life. It has turned out to be a permanent fix for me. You know it beats surgery any day. Dr. Stokes and the staff treated me like I was part of the family, so to speak. We all got to be pretty close. An overall great experience.

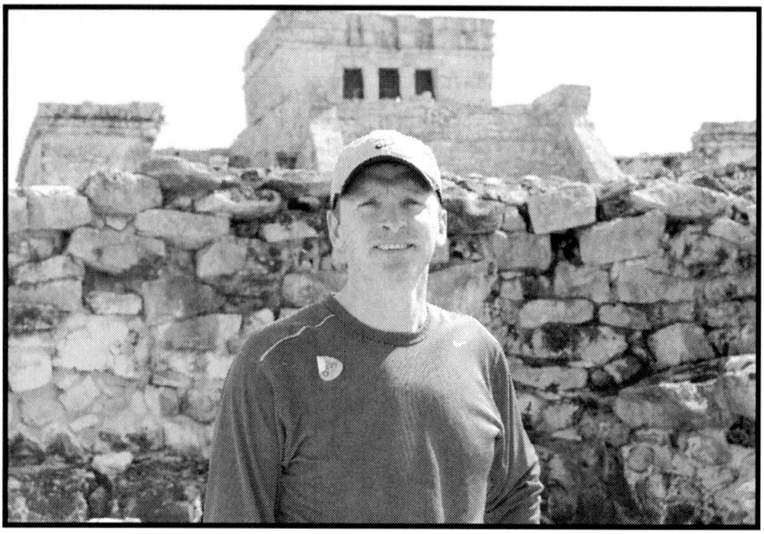

A recent picture taken of me while doing research in Mexico. I am constantly exploring ancient healing rituals including the use of native herbs to better help my patients. Many traditional treatments are quickly being replaced by prescription drugs despite them being more safe and effective. -Dr. Stephen Stokes

Introduction

The Journey

During the 5 years it took me to write this book, I involuntarily went on a life changing journey. I watched helplessly as my back pain worsened and eventually developed into a chronic pain disorder. It took over my entire life and destroyed my health. It forced me to question everything I had learned in school about treating pain. Fortunately, this story has a happy ending, I did get better and the experience opened my eyes to the body's innate ability to heal.

In the early days of trying to help myself I would read hundreds of medical journals every month and speak with doctors from all over the country about my pain. I found myself repeating therapies and protocols because the "experts" said it was the right thing to do. These treatments did not help and most of them made me worse. In retrospect, I now realize this is the greatest injustice we can do to ourselves, ignoring our "gut instinct." As my physical diagnosis professor once remarked,

The retroscope is always 20/20. -Dr. Norman Kettner

Many doctors write about pain but have never experienced it for themselves. They are theorists, who prescribe text book recipes for patient symptoms. I remember being told that I just needed to exercise my back. No pain, no gain I was reminded. This turned out to be horrible advice that rapidly advanced my journey into the world of chronic pain. Today with the research of scientists like Stuart McGill, of the University of Waterloo, we know that strengthening the spinal muscles through exercise actually can lead to an increase occurrence of low back pain. How many times have we heard that all you need to do for back pain is exercise? As you make your own way to recovery always remember that nothing has more credibility than your personal experience. Don't be misled into doing the same thing over and over when you "know" it's wrong.

The definition of insanity is repeating the same action over and over expecting a different outcome. -Albert Einstein

Slowly I got better gaining the confidence and creditability to tell my story. In the last decade I have used this experience to guide thousands of patients towards living a pain free life. There is never one way and never a single solution. Patients, including myself, who have succeeded did so because they never gave up the hope to be better. They were convinced that tomorrow would be a better day. As my dad always would say,

Never give up, never ever give up! -Doug Stokes

So I watch my patients regain their health and in every case there came a point where they turned inward, stopped fighting the condition and allowed innate to take over. This is what researcher William Collinge calls the "turning point." Take a look at the diagram on the top of the next page. Healing is represented as a wavy line with a series of ups and downs but there is a point that marks the shift to higher highs and an upward trend. This is the turning point that we all strive to achieve when trying to overcome any health problem. It is (should be) the goal of all healers to get a patient to this place.

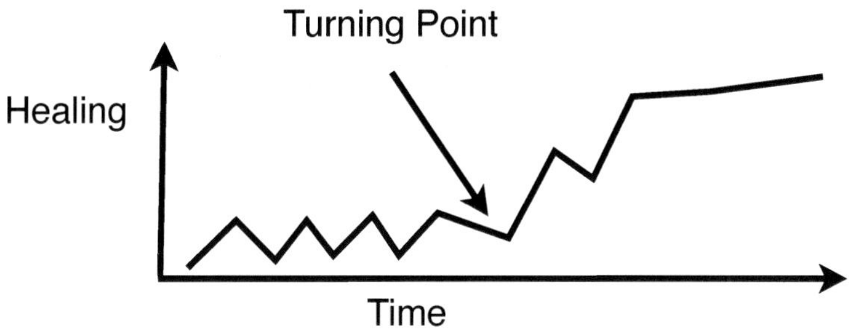

Throughout this book I will present methods for removing obstacles that may be standing in your way of reaching this critical place. By following my instructions you will connect to the Universal Power that creates everything. It is this power, the same power that created your body, that will heal your body. Your innate intelligence is the conduit that can connect you to these higher levels of potential.

In traveling this path you are following in the traditions of the early alchemists. It is well known among all esoteric societies that the transmutation of lead to gold or the "philosophers stone" was a metaphor for the elevation of soul. It is impossible to experience pain and healing without undergoing change. Be prepared you may end up a completely different person.

The Early Years

I have always been healthy and I never feared getting sick. As a young man growing up in St. John's Newfoundland Canada, I was exposed to many harsh elements. If you have never been to St. John's it can easily be described as the city on the edge of the Earth. Picture a harbor surrounded by high cliffs. A city that is constantly beaten by the icy winds blown off wandering icebergs as they make their way down from the North Pole only to get melted by the warm waters of the Gulf Stream. The result of this collision is rain, snow and sleet. St. John's summers are measured in weeks, not months. I grew up there, in this harsh climate. I played rugby against the sailors from the passing ships, scuba dove in the whale invested waters of Conception Bay and ate the traditional diet consisting of salted beef and potatoes. Not much grows in Newfoundland and everything is imported. Fresh fruit and vegetables are a rarity. Still in spite of these facts my constitution was very strong and I was rarely sick as a child. Things always just seemed to come easy for me despite the less than perfect environment. I never had to work very hard at anything. I did good in school, excelled in sports and succeeded at everything I did.

I guess things were a little too easy because at 23 years old I had been in and out of several university programs with nothing to show for my efforts. I would notoriously switch majors mid year, lose credits and in some cases not even show up for the final exams. I just wasn't interested. My father recognized I was having trouble and offered me a job running one of his shopping centers. At the time this was a blessing that gave me some direction. I packed up my new wife Danielle, young son Micheal and set out for Amherst, Nova Scotia. I was excited to be starting over in a new place. I was full of energy, healthy and knew absolutely nothing about anything.

Life in the small town was good and the job allowed me extra time to develop hobbies, one was martial arts. I began training in my backyard and before long I attracted local group of university students that would come over to workout. Although I had practiced traditional forms of martial arts in the past, they all seemed to be lacking continuity. Judo, for example was great for fighting on the ground, boxing had powerful punches, Muay Thai was all kicks and elbows. Each system had strengths but when taken out of it's environment was exposed to weaknesses. I became bored with the traditional martial art systems and started to combined techniques. This was more than 20 years ago, before the current trend of mixed martial arts and ultimate fighting events. By taking a bit of boxing and blending it with kicks and wrestling, I created an effective system of self defense that was more useful than each technique when used on it's own. A style that was not bound by any one system but instead dependent entirely on flowing with the opponent. I named it Budoshin Jitsu, which translates as the way of the warrior. I didn't know it at the time but it was this out of the box thinking that would eventually allow me to create a more effective system to heal my patients. Using the best techniques from many different approaches to form an entirely new and more effective approach was first made famous by martial art legend Bruce Lee. Although I no long practice martial arts, Bruce Lee's philosophy has stayed with me to the present day.

Absorb what is useful - Bruce Lee

Before long I had quite a following and we moved this grass roots movement to the local YMCA. Budoshin Jitsu became quite an attraction even getting a few articles in the local newspaper. My journey into martial arts only lasted 5 years but it sparked an interest inside of me to learn human anatomy. As I struggled to understand the biomechanics of joint locks, knockout strikes or nerve pressure points, I fell in love with biology. Since I lived across the street from the local university I had access to a huge amount of reference material. Soon, I was spending more time studying medical textbooks and less time teaching martial arts. I remember everyday driving through the campus on my way to work and thinking to myself, those lucky kids, walking around drinking coffee and not having to go to work, what a great life. Then one day on my way to work, I just turned off the highway and into the university admissions office. I quit my job that very day and went back to school full time as a biology major at Mount Allison University.

At the time I really didn't know what I would do with this education. I thought about being a teacher or maybe working in research. My dad, being the ever supportive father, asked me if I knew anything about chiropractic. Turns out he had hurt his back on several occasions while lifting weights and found great relief when a chiropractor adjusted his spine. Dad told me that a chiropractors were a doctors who never prescribe drugs, by choice but instead used their hands to fix people. I started looking into chiropractic and the more I learned, the more interested I became. Chiropractic seemed like the ultimate healing profession, sort of like the Budoshin Jitsu of medicine. The best chiropractic school in North America was located just outside of St. Louis, Missouri. I applied and was accepted to Logan College of Chiropractic. I packed up my family (again), sold my little farmhouse across from the university and moved from Canada to Chesterfield, MO. USA.

Chiropractic School

Did I mention I was never sick? I continued to carry this feeling of strength and vitality with me throughout my 20's and 30's. Even while studying disease and pathology at Logan College, I always felt distant from the information because I was in such perfect health. Eventually be my personal experience with chronic pain would bridge the gap between being just technician or becoming a doctor.

My time spent at Logan College was intense. Instead of a normal university program where you are tested once or twice a semester, Logan College tested every week. Many of these exams were oral and they were conducted without notice in front of the entire class.

Mr. Stokes could you please retrace the biological pathway a red blood cell takes as it leaves and then returns to the heart... Mr. Stokes? Please sir, could you stand up and address the class?

Insane stress. There was nowhere to hide and if you didn't know your stuff you would get called out. Frequently students would break down in class and have panic attacks. Looking back it was complete madness. I would attend school all day from 9 am to 4 pm and then have to study from about 7 pm until midnight just to keep up. This went on for just over 4 years! Try to balance this with any type of family life and you can see the conflicts. As my first year at Logan ended, so did my first marriage. Later I learned this sort of collateral damage was common. More than 30% of my married classmates had a divorce while at Logan College. No one should have to choose between career and family. As it turned out I never had to because my wife decided for me. Like I mentioned, after less than a year of student life she left, taking the children, the car, and the silverware. It was a tough time for me but I decided to stay and endure. In the end it would be the right decison. Now more than ever I felt purpose in my life. I had paid a great price to be at Logan College and through that sacrifice I was determined to evolve.

In becoming a doctor of chiropractic I developed the unique skill of correcting spinal subluxations. When spinal joints get injured they can move slightly out of alignment and stop functioning correctly. The correct term for this is a spinal subluxation but the medical community calls it by names like spondylolisthesis, facet syndrome, lumbago, sprains and strains. This condition can pinch or irritate surrounding nerves. A subluxation can stress a spinal disc causing it to herniate and produce the dreaded sciatica.

I had seen the benefits to correcting subluxations while working in the student clinic. People would crawl in and literally leave standing up straight without pain. A chiropractor is the only physician by law that is trained to diagnose and correct a spinal subluxation. Your spine should be checked regularly for subluxations just like you would go to a dentist to keep your teeth healthy. Chiropractic is an essential part of keeping your body healthy before you get sick and that is why it is so unique and needed in todays profit driven medical system. This best approach to health is not a better drug but instead not getting sick in the first place.

It was around this time, perhaps half way through my schooling, that a classmate, Joe Rogers, invited me to have dinner with his girlfriend's family. Her dad was Dr. Mike Fiscella, a local chiropractor with a completely different way of correcting subluxations. He didn't use the traditional bone adjusting protocols I was learning in school. Joe told me Dr. Fiscella rarely even touched the vertebra to correct spinal alignment. I was skeptical but like all students I couldn't afford to turn down the free dinner. With a smart ass know-it-all attitude I headed out fro my free dinner.

What I experienced that evening was something that would forever change the way I viewed chiropractic. After the very best Italian cooking I had ever tasted (this still holds true today) Dr. Fiscella, his daughter Tammy (also a chiropractic student), Joe and myself all went down to his basement. There was a chiropractic table, some basic therapy machines and one of his neighbors waiting patiently to get treated. This was Dr. Fiscella's "Sanctum Santorum".

The first thing Dr. Fiscella does is he turns to me, puts his hand on my shoulder and in his Mid Western, Italian drawl he says,

Muscles move bones, bones don't move muscles. Unless you balance the muscles you will never completely cure the problem.

From the corner of my eye I see the neighbor nodding in agreement as he is taking off his shirt. Muscles? What? Remember I had just spend several years being taught traditional chiropractic methodology, that bones are everything and that the bones move the muscles. As a chiropractor I had developed a love affair with moving bones. This muscle talk was straight out blasphemy! I snarled in protest but unmoved by my rudeness, Dr. Fiscella just smiled and proceeded to treat his neighbor. I watched in disbelief as he completely eliminated all the man's pain in less than 10 minutes without a single pop or crack. There was no chiropractic adjustment preformed but still when Dr. Fiscella was finished the patient reported complete relief and amazingly the subluxation was gone. I was speechless, well not completely, I managed to ask, "Where do I sign up?"

The more I studied muscles, the more I began to suspect they could be the underlying cause of many spinal subluxations. I started to attended train sessions with Dr. Fiscella and began making regular visits to his St. Louis clinic where I could observe the master at work. His protocols were individualized to the patient's needs. People would show up in pain and Dr. Fiscella would work on them until they were fixed. Sometimes 10 minutes, sometimes an hour. In school, I was being taught to see patients on a treatment program consisting of several times a week for 3-4 weeks and then reevaluate for benefit. With Dr. Fiscella there was no set plan, you asked the patient how they felt after each treatment and then decided if they needed to be seen again. This whole process infatuated me. It was so honest and pure. A big departure from mainstream medicine where patients are treated according to their insurance coverage or ability to pay. Dr. Fiscella's patients really loved the treatments, it felt good and there was very few conditions that never responded within a few sessions. I would hear patients talking in the lobby giving testimonials, laughing, sharing stories about how Dr. Fiscella ended their pain in one or two treatments when no other doctor could. As I started becoming proficient in this treatment style, I learned it was originally developed by a brilliant man, Dr. Raymond Nimmo. I also learned that Nimmo's work was the basis of Janet Travel's secret therapy she used to help President John F Kennedy with his chronic back problem. The only treatment, I might emphasize that helped the President despite his access to the country's best doctors. This was powerful stuff.

Dr. Fiscella remains a strong influence on how I treat patients. Many times when faced with a difficult case I ask myself, "What would Dr. Fiscells do?". I have never met a more sincere, dedicated physician and I owe him my career. Dr. Fiscella also helped me after my wife left with some great advice. One day when I was working at his clinic (painting ceiling tiles) he noticed I was a little depressed and he handed me two movie tickets. You see Dr. Fiscella would always send patients free movie tickets on their birthdays so he always had some on hand. He gives me the tickets and said, "Steve, girls love the movies." Just like that I was back in the dating scene. Thanks Mike.

Moving Around

After graduation I spent my first year out of school working as an associate doctor in Battle Creek, Michigan. It was an opportunity to get experience and make some much needed cash. I joined the prestigious practice of Dr. Prebish. We would work 6 days a week seeing over one hundred patients a day. Treating that amount of people was hard work and required spending all day bent over a chiropractic adjusting table. We usually split the patient load between us but when Dr. Prebish took his family on vacation to Ireland, I was the only doctor. One hundred visits in a single day was extreme chiropractic but somehow I got through it. During this time I started noticing a small tingle in my lower back. Not much of a problem just a strange sensation that something was different or "out of whack" in that area. I never paid any attention to it and just kept on working. At the time I was making good money and running on adrenalin. Over the years this tingle in my back would return, sometimes after a heavy workout, a tough day at the office or strangely enough, when I was under stress. The last part was unacceptable to me because despite my extensive training in the physiology of stress I refused to believe I could ever be effected. Stress disorders were for the weak, the sick or at the very least, it was for a patient. I am a doctor after all. So I kept pushing myself and I mean pushing hard. I stayed with Dr. Prebish for exactly one year. It was a great time in my life with many fond memories. If ever in Battle Creek, make sure you get adjusted by Dr. Prebish, he is a true master of what he does and a man of the highest integrity (and a killer golf swing).

While in Battle Creek I married my best friend Katherine Park who I met while at school in St. Louis. We decided to move to Florida and be close to her aging parents. Things were picking up for me, I was very busy and that little tingle in my back seemed a million miles away. My back would hurt from time to time but then quickly disappear. The pain never stayed around very long so I wasn't concerned. We left the cold weather in Battle Creek and headed south for Cape Coral, Florida.

After passing the Florida State chiropractic exam Katherine and myself opened our first clinic together, Primary Care Chiropractic, located on San Carlos Blvd in Fort Myers, Florida. The office was small, only 550 square feet and was attached to a gas station. It was so unusual that other doctors frequently stopped in just to see if it was real. Patients would run in and get an adjustment while they were filling up with gas. I learned how to be very fast and efficient without sacrificing quality. We started helping people and I began to grow in many ways, gaining confidence as a doctor and attracting tougher cases. I think the universe works that way. When you master one thing it starts sending you other opportunities. I would say at this point I had mastered the art chiropractic. I do not mean I was better than everyone else but I had mastered the skills and reached my maximum ability to help people with that modality. Honestly, I was getting a little bored. I saw the same people everyday, non complicated low back and or neck pain and occasionally I would get a headache or a tennis elbow. Most people would get a couple of treatments and the pain went away. Occasionally I would see them in a few months if it came back. Yes, it usually came back but it was not chiropractic's fault. I remember what my supervising doctor told me in student clinic,

Patients are always in a hurry to get back to the things that got them sick in the first place.

So after 5 years of chiropractic school, multiple state and national examinations, I was essentially settling in. Things were good and I was happy. Everything seemed to be in place however I still was lacking the one important quality that all healers require, a personal experience. Regardless of how successful I was there would still remain a disconnect between the patient and myself. After all I had never really been sick and I certainly never had any major problems with my back. Although unfair, I always considered my patients to be weak. They just need to take better care of themselves I thought. They needed more exercise, to lose weight or just stop feeling sorry for themselves. I known this sounds horrible but it was how I felt. Of course the Universe was listening and saw an opportunity to teach me a lesson that would ultimately make me a better doctor.

Adventures In Chronic Pain

It was great day. Katherine and I had gone to the local high school to run track. We did this a lot and enjoyed the opportunity to exercise together in the beautiful Florida sunshine. There was always a variety of people there, a mix of school kids, soccer moms and ex-athletes like myself. We were just finishing up our normal jog when I decided to run the stairs. I guess I thought I was back in my old glory days playing for the Swilers rugby club in Newfoundland. Whatever I was thinking on that day my body had a different agenda. I ran up and down the bleacher stairs for 30 minutes, twisting, jumping and torquing my spine. This felt so good I decided to go home and lift weights for about another hour. The main exercise I did was the dead lift. In this movement you grab a 7 foot steel bar with 315 pounds balanced on it's ends and slowly pull it off the floor to waist height. One swift expression of perfect human biomechanics. "Wow", I thought, "I am really strong, maybe I should start teaching martial arts again?" This would be the very last time in my life I would experience that overwhelming feeling of invincibility. The tingle in my back remained quiet for the remainder of the day.

The next morning I opened my eyes at 6:00 am and I could not get out of my bed to go to the bathroom. The anticipated tingle had no shown itself, in it's place was a severe, tearing sensation that ran across my back and down into my buttocks. It felt like I had broken my spine and I mean this in the most literal sense. Even the slightest movement caused a jolt of electricity to shoot from my spine into my right leg. I slid slowly off the bed and onto the floor. I began to crawled, on my hands and knees to the bathroom, every motion met with an uncontrollable twitching of my lumbar and pelvic muscles. When I got to the toilet, I grabbed the bowl and then the wall. Slowly I crept up, inch by inch, until I got on the toilet seat. "Oh my God," I thought, "What have I done?" My wife called out, "Honey you okay?" She had never seen me in pain like that before. I was in shocked but at that time I was not afraid. The fear would come later, when I learned the extent of the damage I had inflicted on myself.

Somehow I managed to take a hot shower get dressed and drive to my office. I started seeing patients and survived the morning. I was thinking all I needed was to stretch out a little, and loosen up. I even considered maybe going back to the track and doing a little jog. This is how out of touch I was with what was going on. I decided to strap myself to a spinal traction table and crank it open. This table, in case you are not familiar with traction, looks like a medieval torture rack. You lie on your stomach, secure the ankles down with leather straps and slowly split the table in half. As it opens up, while you are holding onto a metal bar, the spinal vertebra are forced apart and the muscles are stretched beyond normal capacity. The theory is to restore normal muscle length by forcing them into position. I did this for maybe 20 minutes and when I was finished it was impossible to get off the table. I was in extreme pain and I had tears in my eyes. I was paralyzed. My wife called some people from the gas station to come over and help me up and into my car. I had to be carried because my legs were numb and the muscles were not working. I laid down in the back seat of the car and Katherine drove us home. So much for needing a little stretch.

I remained in bed for several days, unable to work, feed, bathe or look after myself. This, I thought, is what it is like to be disabled. The days became weeks and to my surprise the pain did not go away. Weeks became months and slowly. Little by little, God granted me a small bit of relief. He knew I was approaching my limit. The pain became tolerable but it never went away. Whenever I tried to regain a little bit of my lost life, exercising, dancing or fishing, the injury would teach me a lesson about who was in charge. Months turned into years and finally I understood what had happened to my spine and yes, now, I was afraid. The diagnosis was a torn L5/S1 lumbar spinal disc that had set off a series of neurological events in my brain to cause a chronic pain syndrome. You can call this fibromyalgia, chronic fatigue syndrome or reflex sympathetic dystrophy it does not matter what you name it, the prognosis was poor and any sort of recovery was unlikely. For me this was simply unbelievable.

So I made a promise to myself that I would learn how pain worked and I set out to overcome it. Up to this point everything I had studied in school was not working for my condition but I was just getting started. Finally, I had being given the precious gift, the one missing element that is essential to becoming a great healer, empathy. It was time for me to see the patient's journey through my own eyes.

Desire is the starting point of all achievement, not a hope, not a wish, but a keen pulsating desire which transcends everything. -Napoleon Hill

Getting The Tools

I started looking for answers, turning over the stones I once never noticed. My first stop was acupuncture. I would spend 2 years studying and eventually became a fellow of the International Academy of Medical Acupuncture under Dr. John Amaro. He was the first person to teach me that a doctor should treat the patient and not the disease. During my training whenever I questioned acupuncture treatment methods Dr. Amaro would say,

The frog in the well knows not of the great ocean.

This is my favorite quote and of course Dr. Amaro was correct. I continued my journey out of the well. I helped hundreds of patients with acupuncture but failed to get relief myself. I was jaded and angry. I decided I would never practice acupuncture again and I threw away all my books and needles. Of course acupuncture had not failed. It works, just like it has worked for thousands of years but I was not ready. Fortunately in these hard times my wife Katherine was always there to encourage me to keep searching and not forget about the frog in the well.

I started intense, obsessive research. Neurology, physiology, anatomy, pathology, I was constantly learning and consulting with specialists. Later, I realized this was the exact opposite of what I needed to do. I learned the hard way that,

A specialist is a doctor who knows more and more about less and less.

These guys, in my experience turned out to be complete idiots. Every specialist said something different from the last one. After a few thousand dollars I realized they didn't have a clue about how I could heal my pain. One even suggested traction! I realized they were not even listening to me. My recover would be up to me and no one else.

Then a friend suggested I attend a presentation by a Canadian chiropractor, Dr. Ted Carrick. I had nothing to lose at this point so I was agreed. Dr. Carrick is the creator of what is now called functional neurology, also known as brain based therapy. Dr. Carrick's treatments are able to activate specific areas of the brain that are responsible for healing. In preparing for the seminar my friend gave me a video of a PBS documentary of Dr. Carrick treating a Parkinson patient with a hand tremor. After about 2 minutes of therapy the patient's tremor stopped. He never once touched the patient's hand. What was going on here? I had to understand the mechanism, it seemed like a magic trick.

Turns out I would spend many years studying with the Carrick Institute, attending weekend seminars, learning how the brain worked and realizing the importance of something called, the central mechanism. This is a very extensive and complicated topic that can take a lifetime of study to fully appreciate but let me give you a summary. Everything in the body is controlled by the brain and spinal cord. This is known as the central nervous system (CNS). It is impossible to successfully treat any type of chronic condition without directly altering the CNS. Let me give you an example. A patient complains of writers cramp. This means whenever they try to write the fingers curled up and cramp. Normally, therapy would be focused on treating the hand including the surrounding muscles, joints and nerves. A traditional treatment approach would be therapy directed at stretching the hand, home exercises and maybe some ultrasound over the sore hand muscles. In contrast, a physician who practices functional neurology would first test the patient to see if the CNS was malfunctioning. In other words, is the problem in the hand or is the problem in the part of the brain that controls the hand?

Through a series of tests it is possible to pinpoint not only the existence of a central problem but also the exact location in the brain where the lesion exists. The clinician then formulates a treatment plan to correct the brain imbalance which stabilizes the CNS. Of course not everybody with writers cramp has a brain based dysfunction, most cases are simply some form of overuse syndrome, but for those patients who do not respond, functional neurology provides a permanently correction. Research shows that in the majority of chronic conditions there is usually at least one brain lesion present. Here is a simple test that checks for a one of these problems.

Sit in a chair and extend both your hands out in front of you. Now close your eyes and slowly try to touch the tip of your nose, one hand at a time. If you have trouble finding your nose or you miss your nose then you may have a brain based condition. It is important to resolve this dysfunction in addition to treating any symptoms you maybe experiencing, otherwise the problem may keep coming back.

Studying the works of Dr. Ted Carrick was like stepping through the looking glass. Never again would I examine a patient the same. I was starting to realized the complexities of treating chronic pain and that there was no simple, one size fits all solution. For me it was sort of like finding out there was no Santa Clause but at least I knew I was on the right path. I continued studying the brain and functional neurology. Soon I was helping more and more patients who had been told there was nothing that could be done for them. The clinic started becoming a place of hope. People were getting excited. I often heard patients talking in the waiting room, "I can move my foot after 5 years" or "I was unable to smell but this morning for the first time since I can remember, I could smell my wife making coffee." This was powerful stuff. I gained a reputation among other physicians for helping people with idiopathic conditions.

Idiopathic is Doctor talk for, "We really have no clue what is going on."

The patient cases were unique and the days never boring. For the first time in my career I was getting referrals from local medical doctors. Of course it was not because they had so much faith in my methods but rather they simply had no idea what else to do for these patients. I think they got tired of not being able to help these patients and just wanted them out of their clinics. It is the craziest thing but once I started helping these tough cases the medical community stopped referring them to me. It was just to much for their egos. Hard to believe but very true, I am sorry to say. Of course at the time I was not completely honest myself. Little did anyone know at that time I was hiding a big secret. Dr. Stokes the super doc who helped all these people was personally suffering from severe chronic pain. I have a sense of humor and so the irony would have been funny in a Monty Python sort of way except that the pain was so devastated I did not think I could continue living with it. Here I was, helping so many people but still unable to fix myself. I started praying several times a day asking the universe "why?" I became paranoid and started to think I was being punished for something I had done in a past life or maybe this life. I had no idea what was going on but it seemed to be a very cruel joke. Luckily my faith pulled me through those hard times. I would say to anyone who feels they are in a hopeless situation, hang on, God will never give you more than you can endure. Pray, meditate, chant, do whatever you must but hang on and if you feel yourself losing grip ask for help. There is no shame in needing help, we are all one being and what happens to one effects us all.

So I held on and then when I was at my lowest suddenly the universe finally responded. At the time I was studying vertigo and the use of balance boards for treatment. While looking online to buy some of these boards for my clinic I came across the Belgau Balance Platform. The ad stated the device was for improving memory and brain function. It never said anything about balance. Eureka, this guy was using functional neurology and not even aware of it. Here was the connection. The part of the brain that controls balance is called the Cerebellum. In addition to balance the cerebellum also regulates nerve signals coming from the spinal muscles into the brain's pain centers. In fact, it turns out the Cerebellum helps to regulate just about every nerve signal coming into the brain. It acts like a neurological amplifier and has the ability to increase or decrease signals thereby assigning priority. I observed the following demonstration.

A stuttering child trained on the Belgau Balance Platform for 10 minutes then was given a random page of Shakespeare to read out loud. Not a fumble, not a single word was misspoken. This was after only 10 minutes.

If the Cerebellum could be accessed that easily maybe balance training could help me heal my back pain? I bought several Belgau Platforms and started working on my balance. I also bought several pieces of 2x4 lumbar and created balance beams in my back yard. I added hand movements, like juggling and touching my nose, while I balancing to further stimulate the

Cerebellum. I tried to balance with one eye closed, in bare feet and eventually by walking backwards. Anything I could think of to increase the intensity. My neighbors must have thought I was training for the circus. Many days when I got home from work I found the local kids in my back yard messing around on my equipment. Other adults in the community were laughing behind my back, "There goes that crazy chiropractor again." My wife remained supportive. She didn't care what people thought because for the first time in years she was seeing improvement in my condition. Not only did I learn to juggle but I also taught all my friends. To this day I display my original Belgau Balance Platform in my office alongside my degrees as a reminder to think outside the box.

After 3 weeks of this specialized rehabilitation my pain reduced dramatically and my function started to return. I was getting excited and decided to have another MRI scan of my back. It showed no change in the protruding spinal disc between L5 and the Sacrum. I was upset with these results. The back was still injured but I was feeling better because my body was better able to deal with the problem. I knew if I wanted a full recovery I would needed to get that disc off my spinal nerve. Although I was definitely in less pain I knew the longer the nerve was compressed by the disc the greater my chances of permanent damage. At this point I had two choices available, spinal surgery or wait until the protrusion degenerated naturally and hope it did not kill the nerve in the process. Neither sounded very promising and since I was starting to feel better I decided to hold off on surgery. I told myself I would wait 6 more months and if nothing changed I would get the surgery. The countdown had started.

Every time I ask a question to the Universe, one way or another I receive an answer. I just pray on the problem and ask for help. This is the most important part, you must acknowledge you need help. You must surrender your ego. Prayer is not difficult, it's just thinking while you are in a very relaxed state. I say to myself, "How can I solve this problem?", then I relax, breath deeply and clear my mind. Who am I asking? I don't know maybe it is

Jesus, Allah, Buddha or maybe my prayers are just an exercise in self fulfillment. I just don't know but someone always responds.

The man who thinks that he is receiving response to his prayers does not know that the fulfillment comes from his own nature, that he has succeeded by the mental attitude of prayer in waking up a bit of this infinite power that is coiled up inside of himself. -How To Know God by Patanjali

Prayer works but if religion and faith are uncomfortable terms for you then just use the accepted scientific name, meditation. If you ask with sincerity and focused intent you will always get a response. Again the surrender is essential. You will not be able to hear a response if you do not think you need help. Trust me, I learned this lesson the hard way.

Ask, and it shall be given you; seek, and ye shall find; knock, and it shall be opened unto you: -Matthew 7:7

This has been a reoccurring truth in my life. Anyone who claims to be a healer and does not submit to a higher power is just a mechanic. The more you learn about science, the further away from spirituality you will be pulled, until ultimately you will find yourself sitting on God's knee. There comes a point where all the data and research will point to the same place, regardless if you are a person of science or religion. We all end up being students of faith. There is a very powerful little book,

The Law of Success by Paramahansa Yogananda

This book is only 34 pages long but it teaches you how to listen to the Universe. Here is a story that illustrates my point about listening to what God is trying to tell you.

The Drowning Man
A fellow was stuck on his rooftop in a flood. He was praying to God for help. Soon a man in a rowboat came by and the fellow

shouted to the man on the roof, "Jump in, I can save you." The stranded fellow shouted back, "No, it's OK, I'm praying to God and he is going to save me." So the rowboat went on. Then a motorboat came by. "The fellow in the motorboat shouted, "Jump in, I can save you." To this the stranded man said, "No thanks, I'm praying to God and he is going to save me. I have faith." So the motorboat went on. Then a helicopter came by and the pilot shouted down, "Grab this rope and I will lift you to safety." To this the stranded man again replied, "No thanks, I'm praying to God and he is going to save me. I have faith." So the helicopter reluctantly flew away. Soon the water rose above the rooftop and the man drowned. He went to Heaven and when he finally got his chance to discuss this whole situation with God, he exclaimed, "I had faith in you but you didn't save me, you let me drown. I don't understand why!" To this God replied, "I sent you a rowboat, a motorboat and a helicopter, what more did you expect?"

So I am wondering about this disc in my back and I am seriously thinking it looks like surgery because I have to get the pressure off the nerve and there is just no other way to do that. I am praying, meditating and listening. Suddenly my phone rings and there is a doctor that I have never heard of on the other end of the line asking me if I am interested in a job. I already had a successful practice so why would I want to go work for someone else? I don't know what made me do this but I get into my car and drive down to his clinic. The sign on the door read,

The Back Pain Institute
Dr. Robert Wootton, DC
VAX-D Disc Therapy

I was greeted by a doctor is in his 70's wearing a blue physicians jacket which I thought was weird because they are usually white. He talks really slow with a southern accent and he tells me his entire practice is focused on repairing damaged spinal discs without any drugs or surgery. At this point the doctor has no idea that I have a damaged disc and it is the first time we have ever met. Here is what he says to me,

You see here Dr. Stokes, well It's all about VAX-D

As he spoke the doctor stared right through me and fixed his gaze upon a before and after MRI hanging behind me on the view box. The films clearly showed a lumbar spinal disc that had apparently healed, completely. The doctor continued...

It stands for vertebral axial decompression, VAX-D for short. Dr. Stokes, I specialize in the treatment of disc problems in the low back.

He grabs an old bone model of the lumbar spine and palms it between his two hands

This is a model of two vertebrae in the low back. These are the bumps you feel down your back called spinous processes. The spinal canal is where the spinal cord goes down through the spine like a telephone cable from the brain and the nerves branch off between the vertebrae. The disc is a pad between the vertebrae that holds the vertebrae together and acts like a shock absorber. It consists of a ring of cartilage that contains the nucleus, which is a spongy cushion that bears your weight. If this cartilage ring stretches out or breaks down, it can bulge or herniate into the spinal canal and press against the spinal cord nerves causing stenosis of the spinal canal. The VAX-D treatment creates a powerful vacuum in the disc that draws in bulges and herniations and stimulates repair cells to heal the disc. It also draws fluid into the disc to re-hydrate the disc and supply nutrition to the disc. It works like traction, but it is totally different. Traction does not help the disc because when traction pulls on the spine the muscles feel the pull and resist it, so it is always pulling against muscle guarding.

Right, I thought to myself, I learned that the hard way, I almost killed myself on a traction table trying to force my muscle to relax. That was something I wanted no part of.

Now Dr. Allan Dyer is a well-known medical doctor. He was the Minister of health for Ontario, Canada and he also did research that helped invent the heart defibrillator – those paddles that start the heart. He had research that showed if the pull is increased on a logarithmic curve – that's a mathematical formula – the pull is so gradual that the muscles are not aware of the pull, so they stay relaxed. That allows it to pull directly on the disc. If you stretch the disc itself, it is like pulling on the plunger of a hypodermic needle – it creates a powerful vacuum inside the disc. The pressure inside the resting disc is 75 mm Hg. No traction can lower the pressure to 35 mm Hg. With VAX-D I can routinely lower the pressure to 100 mm Hg below 0. That's a powerful vacuum that draws in bulges and herniations and stimulates repair cells that heal the disc. Come with me and let me show you what we are talking about.

We walked into a small room filled with two over sized metal consoles complete with pressure dials, buttons and graph paper print out. Each unit was attached, by what looked like an umbilical cord, to a futuristic looking exam table that was split in the middle. The whole scene was like something you would find in a NASA research department. I remember thinking, there is absolutely no way I am ever getting on that equipment.

You lie face down on the table and this harness goes around your waist and attaches to this post at the foot of the table. There are handles to hold on to or we can use a strap to hold you in place. It pulls for one a minute, releases for a thirty-seconds and then rests for another thirty-seconds. This repeats fifteen times. So, you are on the table for thirty minutes. We start with twenty visits done daily. It is computer operated and it records the pounds of pull of each cycle. It works by air pressure so it is very smooth acting. This is the control knob that sets the pounds of pull, but, no matter how many pounds we set it at, the computer keeps it exactly on the logarithmic curve and that's what makes it work. It's a very high-tech treating table that gets great results in disc problems of the lower back.

He turns a large dial and pushes a yellow button. I hear an air compressor turn on followed by the sound of a piston firing. An alarm bell sounds, "Beep, beep, beep" and the table begins to separate.

See how slowly it moves? It goes slower and slower as it pulls harder and harder. That's the logarithmic increase and the muscles aren't aware of the pull so it is pulling directly on the disc and creating a powerful vacuum that draws in herniations and bulges. Let's go back to my office and have a seat. Now when you first start the treatment your disc is all stretched out. On each pull the disc is drawn in, but in the beginning it goes back out. As you continue the treatments the disc begins to heal and by the time you've had twelve to fifteen treatments the disc begins to hold. Some people feel better in a few treatments when things begin to loosen up, but the average person may not feel any relief at all until they have had about twelve treatments. Then the disc begins to hold and pressure comes off the nerves and they begin to feel better. By the time they have their basic twenty visits they have a fairly strong disc. If you get five or six treatments and stop, you'll lose it all. It's like if you have a cast on a fractured arm and take it off in two weeks it might be strong for a day or two but it will probably break down. If you leave it on for the six to eight weeks that it takes to heal a bone, you'll have a bone that is stronger than the original because the repair cells are the strongest tissue in your body. The same with a disc – once it is healed it is stronger than the original. By the time they have their basic twenty visits 35% of the people are pain free and 45% of the people are better. 15% of the patients don't respond very well. If they don't respond at all we don't go any further. If they go on to thirty visits, they have a stronger disc and 70% of the people are pain free. If they go on to forty visits, 80% of the people are pain free. If they go beyond 40 we can help about 5 or 6% more. So the VAX-D gives a very high potential for improvement for disc conditions of the low back. By comparison, surgery – not that I recommend surgery – surgery helps one out of three cases, and one out of three are worse and one out of three are no better. VAX-D helps eight out of ten. So VAX-D is more than twice as effective as surgery. With surgery you have a list of risk factors like scar tissue buildup, infection, nerve damage, paralysis, and even the anesthesia is a high risk factor. VAX-D is noninvasive so it has none of those risk factors making it far safer than surgery.

He paused, expressionless, waiting for me to comment. Nothing was said, he looked into my eyes, I swear he looked right into my soul. There is about 10 seconds of total silence when finally he makes a slight smile and simply says,

You'll start tomorrow.

There was no mention of hours, contracts or wages. That was it, interview over. I had a new job. We shook hands, I went back to my office and told my wife what happened. I would transfer my current patients to the new office and close Primary Care Chiropractic. I didn't care about going to work for someone else. The Universe was presenting my Guru. Once you get a glimpse of the truth you have to follow it because everything else is just a lie and no matter how attractive or easy that path maybe it is still a lie. In the Book of Secrets, Osho explains to his followers how we must follow the truth despite potential hardships. No matter how easy, the false path will not led to enlightenment.

The Street Light

Late one evening, a man who was walking his dog comes upon another man who is searching the ground under a street light. The passerby asks what he is doing. "I'm looking for my lost keys," says the man searching the ground. "I dropped them on my way home" he says. The passerby offers to help search for the keys, but after several minutes of searching under the street light they have no luck. "Are you sure you dropped them here?" asks the passerby. "Oh, I have no idea if I dropped them here," says the man. "Then why are you only looking under this street light?" "Well…" replies the man, "Because this is where I can see the best.

Finding My Path

Over the next few years I became a master of VAX-D therapy, serving as the medical director for 3 of the states largest, most successful clinics. I oversaw locations in Fort Myers, Naples and West Palm Beach, helping thousands of people avoid back surgery. Everything the wise Doctor Wootton said turned out to be true, for many people VAX-D was nothing short of a miracle. I cannot tell you exactly how many lives I changed but I still occasionally meet someone at the grocery store or at the beach who knows someone that I helped. As for my own back pain, VAX-D removed the pressure on my spinal nerve. That's right, no more nerve compression. Yes, the disc protrusion was corrected with VAX-D but I did not completely recover from my injury. Turns out that when the body is hurting for a long time it changes. It learns to compensate and essentially it rewires. Your pain threshold alters and over time the way your brain runs things is never the same. I have learned from personal experience that the body does not completely repair, instead it heals and there is a big difference. Damaged tissue will never be exactly the same as healthy tissue just like a scar is less mobile. This is not the end of hope for all you pain sufferers, listen to me, I am no longer living a life ruled by pain. Today I am essentially normal but that little tingle in my back has left its mark. It changed who I am. If you are suffering from chronic pain your journey will change you as well. No one gets to stay the same. By following the advice in this book you will learn to heal and regain your life. You will have the tools to make sense of your condition. Life is a beautiful experience but remember it is only by feeling bad we understand what it is like to feel good. So what happened to the rest of my story? Well, it did not end there with VAX-D. Turns out there were more secrets to discover. As my knowledge of how the body heals grew I could no longer only see patients with back pain, soon I was seeing many different types of illnesses. The word was out and I started getting referrals from local medical doctors, massage therapists, physical therapists and acupuncturists. I remember one case where the referral was a patient with Lupus. This is a serious autoimmune disease for which there is no cure. When I called the doctor and told him I was a back pain doctor his response was,

Well, look Doc, she has heard about you from her friends and is convinced you can help besides she is having back pain, so why don't you just give her a crack.

Crack is a slang word used by uneducated people to describe the chiropractic adjustment of a subluxation. To me crack would be a more appropriate slang for the medical doctors treatment, but anyways. I started working on her back and every visit she asked me if I could suggest anything to help with the Lupus. She had heard people in the lobby reporting improvement with all sorts of conditions and figured out that I may have some answers. This was my big chance. I remember exactly what I did for this patient. It was no big deal. I mentioned she may want to try Echinacea, specifically a combination of E. angustifolia and E. purpurea root. This herbal product does not stimulate the immune system but balances it. Since Lupus is an autoimmune disorder I figured it would be a good place to start. That was all I did, nothing else. Her back pain went away in a few treatments and I lost contact with her. I bumped into her at the Publix grocery store 6 months later. She told me her Lupus was under control and she was no longer taking steroids, only Echinacea. I had totally forgotten about the whole thing and had to act like I knew what she was talking about. Later I pulled her chart and realized what she was talking about. I was impressed. I wondered how many more patients I could help if I started to focus on the biochemical aspects of disease.

I dug out my biochemistry textbooks and start to obsessively study metabolic pathways. I contacted one of the top pharmaceutical companies, Roche and they sent me a huge wall chart that showed every chemical reaction produced in the body. This would serve as my initial road map. I studied the mechanisms of disease and pain and how the drugs altered those reactions. I realized quickly that there were many opportunities to influence those reactions using herbs and natural materials. This was exciting and felt like another secret door had opened in my professional life. At first I though I was alone in my research but I soon found an emerging branch of healthcare called Functional Medicine that was publishing studies in this area. It was at this time I discovered Jeffery S Bland, PhD, FACN, CNS. He was the chief science officer for Metagenics. Dr. Bland was publishing research that showed you could make objective changes on many diseases through proper nutritional supplementation. He used the term "nutraceuticals" to distinguish the products he was formulating from the unregulated, untested vitamin market. High blood pressure, diabetes, heart disease, all improved with Dr. Bland's protocols. As I included functional medicine into my treatment plans patients experienced dramatic changes. I became thirsty for more. No longer was I content to just see back pain patients, I wanted to help as many people as possible.

I resigned my position as Medical Director for the Back Pain Institute and left the company. Another doctor who shared my vision, Dr. Gary Goerg joined my quest. Together we set out to create a clinic that would help people suffering from chronic illness and pain. This would be accomplished without using drugs or surgery. I wanted better results than the medical community were getting and I wanted the ability to help anyone that walked in the door. Regardless if you had a sprained ankle or pancreatic cancer, I want to provide help and hope. Dr. Goerg owned a phase contrast microscope and was an expert of nutritional analysis using saliva, urine and blood. We could test our patients initially and then retest at frequent intervals to validate the effectiveness of the treatments. We began to gather a lot of data and

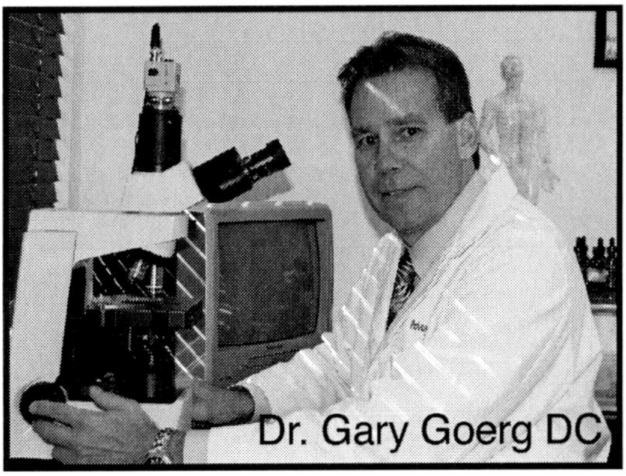

our protocols became more effective. There was no turning back.

The goal was simple, all treatments would help the body in dealing with whatever disease it was experiencing. The names, labels or diagnosis did not matter. I was interested in treating person who had a disease and not a disease that had person. This is a simple idea that has been lost in medicine today. To do this and be successful, I had to look beyond the illness and the labelled diagnosis. I needed to understand how the body worked and then apply treatment that would help the body heal itself. You see the body does a good job at taking care of itself without any intervention from the outside, but if something goes wrong it may then need a little help. I found the best way to do this was with a systemic approach. So I did what I alway did, I asked the Universe for a solution. This time the answer would be me. I had gone on the journey and survived. By retracing my own steps in healing, I could formulated a treatment philosophy and set of effective procedures that worked regardless of the specific diagnosis. There are common elements like inflammation, pain and immune response to all chronic diseases, correcting these problems help the body heal any condition.

At the time this was a hard path to follow. Many physicians consider my model backward thinking. They are obsessed with symptoms and providing drugs to suppress those symptoms without digging deeper to correct the cause. I frequently was criticized by other doctors. Patient's were told not to go and see me or that I was a running some sort of a scam. When blood pressure came down with my treatment the primary doctor would say it was a placebo. Of course he was right. The whole idea was to get the body to heal itself, in a sense the placebo is the most powerful medicine. At the time all this negative feedback really hurt my feelings but eventually I stopped trying to win recognition from the medical community. We played for opposite teams and they were not going to go against the drug companies, there was just too much money at stake.

So the work goes on and along the way some people, "get it" but still many do not and it has become my life's work to preach the truth to those who will listen and to accept those who will not as merely unwilling to acknowledge at this time that they need help.

7 Steps To Innate Healing

Doctors are men who prescribe medicines of which they know little, to cure diseases of which they know less, to human beings of which they know nothing.
-Voltaire

How Medicine Got Sick

Did you watch the news last night? Have you noticed TV commercials advertising drugs to treat things like fibromyalgia, chronic fatigue or irritable bowel syndrome. You couldn't find these disorders mentioned in medical journals 10 years ago but now they have become mainstream. Why is this? Obviously we are sicker today than ever before in the history of our country. The current medical system is not working. Treating the symptoms of disease with suppressive toxicology does not work, it has never worked and people just end up getting sicker, not only suffering from the disease also the side effects of the drugs. This is especially true in the treatment of chronic illnesses. When was the last time you heard about someone taking a drug to cure diabetes or heart disease?

America is not healthier, just better managed.

Allen Roses is vice president of genetics at Glaxo Smith Kline, an international drug company, he stated:

The vast majority of drugs, more than 90% only work in 30 to 50% of the people.

What does that mean? It means that most drugs do not work. Of course people don't talk about this. Patients assume that prescribed drugs work but what they do not realize is that they only have to work some of the time, on some of the people. What's interesting is that the FDA approves these drugs for public consumption when they have such a low rate of success and in many cases will do more damage than good. If you have ever listened to the side effects of the medications advertised during the nightly news it is quite an enlightening experience. The drug companies don't want you to pay attention to the side effects so they show people laughing, dancing and having fun while in the background the announcer's voice reads the fine print. Routinely side effects will include are liver failure, cancer and suicide. Does it seem ironic to you that anti depressant medications can cause a side effect of suicide? Seriously, how is this sort of nonsense allowed by a caring, intelligent government protection agency like the FDA.

In the last 5 years the government has forced the FDA to decrease the amount of time it requires to approve a drug for the market. Why would they do that? Do you think it has anything to do with pressure from the pharmaceutical companies? Of course it does. Every day that a new drug is not approved can cost millions of dollars. So most of these medications get quickly passed and pushed through. No one knows what the long-term effects are of taking prescription medication, especially the FDA, who are the ones endorsing it to the public. Think about how many times have we been told about some new wonder drug only to hear later that it is being pulled from the market or it is involved in some nasty class action suit.

If you are taking more than three prescription drugs it is impossible to predict the side effects caused by the drug interactions. Just ask any high school chemistry teacher and if they are not on the drug companies payroll, they will agree. Ever wonder why the side effects are written on a sheet of paper that comes in the medication package. Why not list them right on the bottle? Not enough room. Besides staring at all those nasty side effects every time you take your pills is bad for business. After all you may start to thinking these things are not so good for you. If you saw those side effects on a bottle of shampoo for your dog you wouldn't use it on the animal but here in "pill nation" educated, caring people give their children Tylenol everyday. Of course it's bubble gum flavored Tylenol, because we want our kids to enjoy taking the medicine. In case you don't know Acetaminophen is the active ingredient in Tylenol. It is found in many other over-the-counter and prescription drugs. Things like painkillers and fever reducers. Now what is interesting is that no one really knows how this stuff works, it just seems to work. They really have no idea of the biochemical pathways involved. The science just doesn't make sense but no one really seems to care. Acetaminophen is so widely used, many mistakenly believe it to be completely harmless. Not true. It is estimated that acetaminophen poisoning results in 56,000 injuries, 25,000 hospitalizations, and 450 deaths every year. Medical professionals (the same groups who prescribe this stuff) have concluded that long-term use, or large doses of the drug can damage the liver, leading to liver failure or even death. The U.S. Acute Liver Failure Study Group found that acetaminophen poisoning is the leading cause of liver failure in the nation, accounting for approximately half of all cases. Some of these instances of liver failure occur even when following the dosage recommendations printed on the bottle.

The drug companies are no different then the tobacco industry. They need to build a client based and customer loyalty from an early age. So they put friendly, cartoon camels on cigarette packaging and as I mentioned earlier, they make Tylenol in bubble gum flavor. Shame on you McNeil Pharmaceutical. This is criminal.

Still none of this matters, business is booming! We have more drugs to treat more diseases than ever before in the history of our country. Drugs to go to sleep, drugs to wake up, drugs to go to the bathroom, drugs to prevent you from going to the bathroom. We are creating disorders and then matching them up with prescription drugs at an alarming rate. It's a monopoly in the most real sense and it is a billion dollar industry. That's billions. Here is what a billion dollars looks like,

$1,000,000,000 (one thousand million dollars)

You have to understand that it's all a bunch of lies. Every year in the United States, according to the groundbreaking 2003 medical report *Death by Medicine*, by Drs. Gary Null, Carolyn Dean, Martin Feldman, Debora Rasio and Dorothy Smith, more than 110,000 people die from prescription drugs. Remember that is from 2003. Centers for Disease Control and Prevention have reported that in the last 10 years there has been a fourfold increase in prescription drug related deaths. So the numbers are obviously much higher today and these are not junkies or people abusing medicine, these are normal people who are taking exactly what the doctor told them to take and they die as a result. How did we ever get so far off purpose from the original Hippocratic Oath taken today by all graduating medical students? The answer is greed.

Hippocratic Oath

I swear to fulfill, to the best of my ability and judgment, this covenant:

I will respect the hard-won scientific gains of those physicians in whose steps I walk, and gladly share such knowledge as is mine with those who are to follow. I will apply, for the benefit of the sick, all measures that are required, avoiding those twin traps of over treatment and therapeutic nihilism.

I will remember that there is art to medicine as well as science, and that warmth, sympathy, and understanding may outweigh the surgeon's knife or the chemist's drug.
I will not be ashamed to say "I know not", nor will I fail to call in my colleagues when the skills of another are needed for a patient's recovery.
I will respect the privacy of my patients, for their problems are not disclosed to me that the world may know. Most especially must I tread with care in matters of life and death.
If it is given to me to save a life, all thanks. But it may also be within my power to take a life; this awesome responsibility must be faced with great humbleness and awareness of my own frailty. Above all, I must not play at God.
I will remember that I do not treat a fever chart, a cancerous growth, but a sick human being, whose illness may affect the person's family and economic stability. My responsibility includes these related problems, if I am to care adequately for the sick.
I will prevent disease whenever I can, for prevention is preferable to cure.
I will remember that I remain a member of society with special obligations to all my fellow human beings, those sound of mind and body as well as the infirm.
If I do not violate this oath, may I enjoy life and art, respected while I live and remembered with affection thereafter. May I always act so as to preserve the finest traditions of my calling and may I long experience the joy of healing those who seek my help.

My favorite line in the oath is,

I will prevent disease whenever I can, for prevention is preferable to cure.

Perhaps they should rework the oath to read,

I will treat symptoms while avoiding the cure because profits are found in management and not the correction of disease.

Today there are more than 105 million Americans experiencing some type of chronic pain or degenerative disease. That's a big number and it eats up more than 70% of all the time doctors spend with patients. These people are suffering, they are miserable and they are not getting better. As a result 3/4's of all US health care dollars are spent on what comes down to disease management. Big money for a low return. American men have a 50% chance of getting cancer and women a 40% chance. Heart disease will kill 1 in 3 Americans. One dollar out of every seven in our economy goes for health care. We are the sickliest nation on earth. Each American spends over $4,000 a year on heath care.

A Real Cure for Chronic Illness

The trend in Medicine today is towards specialization not generality. Doctors are being taught more and more about less and less. If this continues, in the future there will be no general physicians left, only specialists and you cannot compartmentalize the human body, everything is connected. Recently, a close friend of mine complained how he went to his general practitioner to have a wart removed and was referred to a hand surgeon. Completely unnecessary. Even 10 years ago any doctor worth his salt would have been all over that wart. My brother in law is a medical doctor in Canada and he loves to cut, sew, trim and inject. He says it makes him feel like a "real doctor" in an otherwise boring family practice. When I asked him why general doctors are fading out he said they cannot afford the malpractice insurance that would be required to preform all those in office treatments, like removing a wart. People sue and it is not worth stepping outside the box so it becomes easier to just refer out. Passing the buck or the wart, in this case, is becoming the standard within the American and Canadian Medical Associations. Problem is that this system doesn't work so good. You must treat the entire person to heal the entire person. This makes sense because all systems of the body interact with one another. The body is more than just a collection of systems, organs, tissues and fluids that independently breakdown or malfunction. The body is an integrated unit. Health is more than the absence of symptoms. This is why healthcare is failing. It is the movement towards specialization that is leading the decline.

I knew the solution to helping cure disease was a systemic approach and not a symptom approach. This is the first key to success in treating hard cases.

1. Disease and sickness cannot occur in a healthy body where all the systems are working together. Symptoms are a sign that the system is failing. The symptom is not the cause.

Let's say a person is complaining that they have a problem with roaches in their kitchen. So they buy traps and sprays. For a few months the bugs disappear but they eventually return. This cycle continues and the roach problem becomes an accepted part of living in the house. However the cause of the problem is never addressed, which is that the home owners are always leaving opened food containers in the cupboards. Once they start practicing better storage methods the roach problem goes away. So we have to always be thinking about the body as a whole. Here is the second secret in treating sick patients,

2. The body is a self healing organism when all systems are functioning at an optimal level.

This is very powerful, this is huge. There is no mention of drugs or surgery here. Honestly, for most simple problems you do not need a doctor. Your body does a much better job at healing than any modality available. Get the body working correctly and you can heal any disease. This book will guide you towards stimulating your own self healing force, called innate. This will be achieved by systematically evaluating your body systems and correcting current dysfunction. Once all systems are operating effectively innate will take over and do its job.

Of course there are certain conditions that require conventional medicine. It would be foolish to discount allopathic medicine and in certain conditions it is absolutely needed. Dr. Andrew Weil gives the following advice,

Do not seek help from a conventional doctor for a condition that conventional medicine cannot treat, and do not rely on alternative providers for a condition that conventional medicine can manage well. -Andrew Weil, Spontaneous Healing

Dr. Weil continues to make the following distinctions in what allopathic medicine can and cannot do for the patient:

CAN
Manage trauma better than any other system of medicine.
Diagnose and treat many medical and surgical emergencies.
Treat acute bacterial infections with antibiotics.
Treat some parasitic and fungal infections.
Prevent many infectious diseases by immunization.
Diagnose complex medical problems.
Replace hips and knees.
Get good results with cosmetic and reconstructive surgery.
Diagnose and correct hormonal deficiencies.

CANNOT
Treat viral infections.
Cure most chronic degenerative diseases.
Effectively manage most kinds of mental illness.
Cure most forms of allergy or autoimmune disease.
Effectively manage psychosomatic illness.
Cure most forms of cancer.

This book, **Heal Yourself: The 7 Steps To Innate Healing**, was originally a workbook written for my patients. Over the years it has been modified and developed to it's current format. Today, these 7 steps can ignite your own ability to heal regardless of the cause. They are presented in order of importance but you can start anywhere, your final destination will end up being the same. It is not a replacement to conventional medicine and if it seems as I am suggesting such than I am being misunderstood. Rather I suggest that both traditional and non traditional medicine can operate together, each operating within its boundaries to accomplish it's goals.

You don't have to accept your fate and become a statistic. For over a decade I've treated patients who have been unable to find help anywhere else. I've seen thousands of people who were told they had incurable diseases and that the best they could hope for was a lifetime of medications or invasive surgical procedures. These are the patients who fill my office every day, these are the real people whose lives have changed with this information. It is common in my practice to witness patients with serious diseases helped in less than a year. People on diabetes medication with normal blood sugar levels after just six months of following my program. Men and women who were told they needed heart bypass surgery given a clean bill of health from the cardiologist in only 9 months. These so called incurable diseases can be healed through proper diagnosis and treatment. When I accept a patient I am not focused on cost, time or political correctness, only the results. My goal is to educate you, guide you and fix you. Then I expect you to be my patient for life. Once a patient asked me how long they would need to see me and I told them for the rest of their life. I know it seems extreme but it's an honest answer. Once you are better you will need to stay that way. I see some people every week, others once a month and many check in several times a year. All my patients are given an outline of how to live, if a patient chooses to follow, I see them less however if they get off purpose, I see them more frequently. The great thing about the health wagon is it moves slow enough that if you fall off you can always get back on.

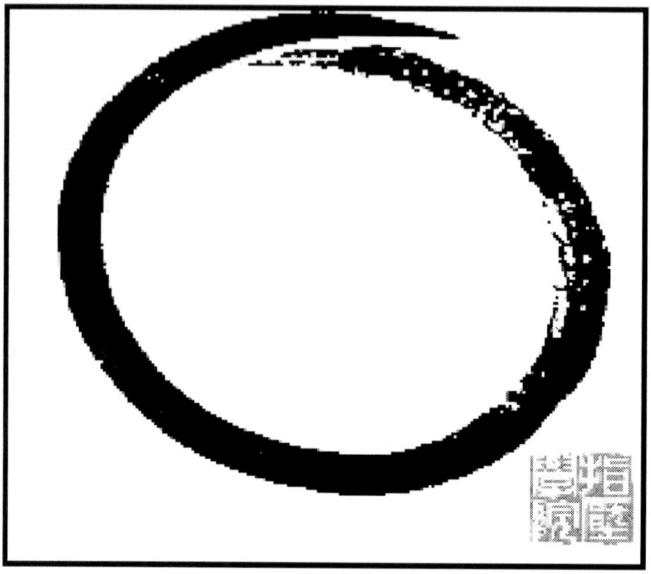

ZEN gives you the discipline, to become a mirror, in such a way that you can reflect that, what is. Everything that you need is perception that not is distorted by thinking. -OSHO

Step One: Relieve Your Pain

Every nerve that can thrill with pleasure, can also agonize with pain.
-HORACE MANN, A Few Thoughts for a Young Man

What Is Pain?

Your nervous system is made up of two parts: the central which is the brain and the spinal cord and the peripheral which contains both sensory and motor nerves. The names make it easy to picture: the brain and spinal cord are the hub, while the sensory and motor nerves stretch out to provide access to all areas of the body. Put simply, sensory nerves send impulses about what is happening in our environment to the brain via the spinal cord. The brain sends information back to the motor nerves, which help us perform actions. It's like having a very complicated in and out box for everything. Let's say you step on a rock. How does a sensory nerve in the peripheral nervous system know this is any different than something like a soft toy? Different sensory nerve fibers respond to different things, and produce different chemical responses which determine how sensations are interpreted. Some nerves send signals associated with light touch, while others respond to deep pressure.

Special pain receptors called nociceptors activate whenever there has been an injury, or even a potential injury, such as breaking the skin or causing a large indentation. Even if the rock does not break your skin, the tissues in your foot become compressed enough to cause the nociceptors to fire off a response. Now, an impulse is heading through the nerve into the spinal cord, and eventually all the way to your brain. This happens within fractions of a second. Your spinal cord is a complex array of bundles of nerves, transmitting all kinds of signals to and from the brain at any given time. It is a lot like a freeway for sensory and motor impulses. But your spinal cord does more than act as a message center: it can make some basic decisions on its own. These "decisions" are called reflexes.

Dorsal Root Ganglion (DRG)

An area of the spinal cord called the dorsal root ganglion (DRG) acts as an information hub, simultaneously directing impulses to the brain and back down the spinal cord to the area of injury. The brain does not have to tell your foot to move away from the rock, because the dorsal horn has already sent that message. If your brain is the body's CEO, then the spinal cord is middle management. Even though the spinal reflex takes place at the dorsal horn, the pain signal continues to the brain. This is because pain involves more than a simple stimulus and response. Simply taking your foot off the rock does not solve all of your problems. No matter how mild the damage, the tissues in your foot still need to be healed.

The Limbic System

In addition, your brain needs to make sense of what has happened. Pain gets catalogued in your brain's library, and emotions become associated with stepping on that rock. When the pain signal reaches the brain it goes to the thalamus, which directs it to a few different areas for interpretations. A few areas in the cortex figure out where the pain came from and compare it to other kinds of pain with which is it familiar. Was it sharp?

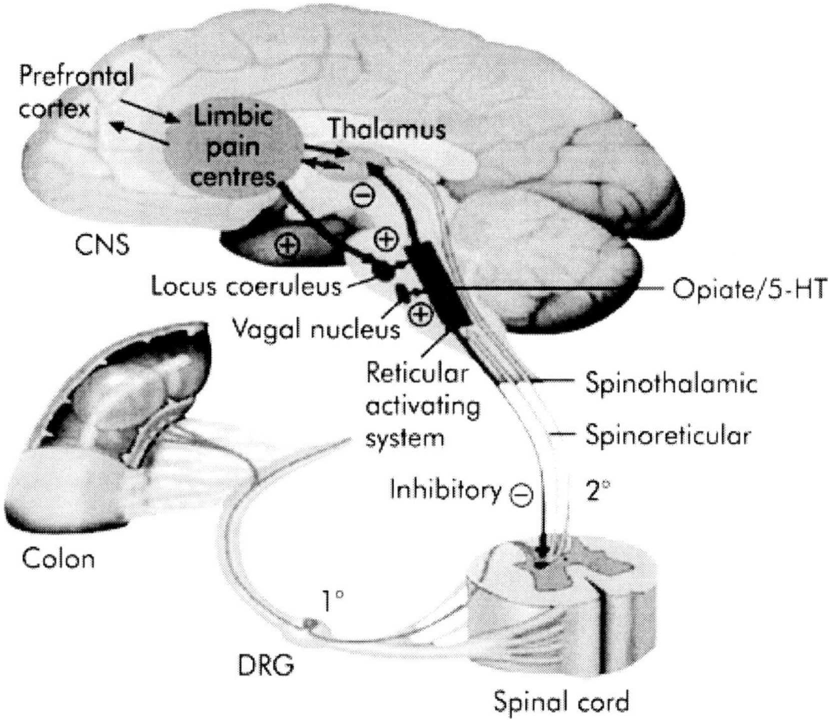

Here is a diagram of the pain pathway. In this example an impulse comes from the colon and travels to the DRG and then on to the Thalamus which is strongly influence by your emotions (Limbic Center). It is easy to explain how stressful emotions can cause constipation in the colon with this model. If the DRG is malfunctioning your brain will think there is a problem with the colon when it maybe perfectly well.

Did it hurt more than stepping on a tack? Have you ever stepped on a rock before, and if so was it better or worse? Signals are also sent from the thalamus to the limbic system, which is the emotional center of the brain. Ever wonder why some pain makes you cry? The limbic system decides. Feelings are associated with every sensation you encounter and each feeling generates a response. Your heart rate may increase, and you may break out into a sweat. All because of a rock underfoot. While it may seem simple, the process of detecting pain is complicated by the fact that it is not a one-way system. It isn't even a two-way system. Pain is more than just cause and effect: it is affected by everything else that is going on in the nervous system. Your mood, your past experiences and your expectations can all change the way pain is interpreted at any given time. How is that for confusing? If you step on that rock after you have a fight with your wife, your response may be very different than it would if you had just won the lottery. Your feelings about the experience may be tainted if the last time you stepped on a rock, your foot became infected. If you stepped on a rock once before and nothing terrible happened to you, you may recover more quickly. You can see how different emotions and histories can determine your response to pain. In fact, there is a strong link between depression and chronic pain.

Acute vs Chronic Pain

In the step on a rock scenario, after your foot healed, the pain sensations would stop. This is because the nociceptors no longer detect any tissue damage or potential injury. This is called acute pain.

Pain that has started recently or has only existed for a short duration (less than 3 months), is known as acute pain.

Acute pain does not persist after the initial injury has healed. The body is still trying to repair the damage and there is a very good chance that you will get better once the process is completed. In some injuries, like ligamentous sprains, this process can take a long time but as long as your body is working towards repairing the problem it can be considered acute pain. Just because it is acute does not mean it is not serious. A fatal car accident, gunshot wound or heart attack are all acute problems. In general, acute pain is the easiest condition to treat because your body will heal as long as you do not irritate or re-injure the area. The traditional medical model is set up for handling acute pain and it is very good at it. Most injury a person will come across throughout life is considered acute. Sometimes, however, pain receptors continue to fire. This can be caused by a disease or condition that continuously causes damage. With arthritis, for example, the joint is in a constant state of disrepair, causing pain signals to travel to the brain with little down time. Sometimes, even without tissue damage, nociceptors continue to fire. There may no longer be a physical cause of pain, but the pain response is the same. This is know as chronic pain and it is very difficult to treat.

Pain that remains for more than 6 months or goes away but returns on occasion is considered chronic pain.

Chronic pain is a monster. These conditions can last forever if not properly treated. Reoccurring migraines, back pain when you sit for too long, neck pain first thing in the morning or a skin condition that never clears up are all chronic problems. If you try to treat them the same way you would treat an acute problem they usually get worse. When a condition changes from acute to chronic the pain switches from being generated at the site of injury to being brain based. In other words the brain changes it's wiring to accept the injury and no longer requires updates from the original damage. This is major because what it means is that once a condition becomes chronic you may still have pain even if the original site of injury get completely mended. It also means that in chronic conditions your body has stopped trying to fix the problem and instead has accepted the injury as permanent.

In chronic pain that DRG we talked about earlier gets switched on and overrides communication to the brain. Once the DRG is switched on it is very hard to turn off. The DRG is like a car alarm that keeps firing even after the threat is long gone. Even powerful pain killing drugs will do little to turn off the DRG once it gets activated. The good news is that the DRG gets all it's information from sensors in the body. These sensors respond to mechanical stimulation, temperature changes and chemical irritation and they only live for a few days before they are replaced by new ones. So this means that even in the worst cases of chronic pain there is hope, your current sensitivity level is not "carved in stone", with the correct treatment the DRG can be deactivated.

Substance P

As we already have seen there is a lot more to pain than just feeling bad. Pain is a whole cascade of chemical signals that cause undesirable reactions in the body. We have heard the saying, "no pain no gain" and I want you to completely wipe that out of your memory. Do not allow yourself to experience pain for very long. The reason has to do with a neuropeptide that is released from the ends of your sensory nerves, called substance P. This chemical responds to pain and inflammation by helping your body make more pain receptors. So you become more aware of pain because your ability to detect it improves. If a person has too much substance P in their system they can become hyper sensitive to pain which will cause normal activities to hurt. This is not psychological pain, this is real and it is one way that our body develops chronic pain syndromes like fibromyalgia. So you have to stop the process of pain before it grows into a bigger problem.

We need to be aware of what is happening when we feel pain and we need to respect the process. Ignoring pain is a bad idea but remember that nothing in the body is ever permanent, there is always a chance to grow new sensors and start healing. There is no such thing as a hopeless case. We have learned about pain in the last 5 years, more than we have known in the last 50. Most doctors just do not have a current understanding of this new neurology and treat chronic problems with acute methods.

The Cause Spinal Pain

Since back pain is perhaps one of the most common conditions experienced by my patients I am going to explain how it is caused. Although there are differences the basic mechanism for back pain is very similar to most other forms of muscular skeletal pain, so many of these terms will apply to conditions like knee pain, tennis elbow and hip problems.

It is important to understand that many things can initiate back pain. It can be physical trauma such as a sports or lifting injury, poor posture, structural problems like a short leg or even pronated feet. All of these things can predispose you to pain. There are also many chemical triggers that can set the pain off. These are the primary focus of functional medicine and include poor nutrition, hormone imbalances and abuse of drugs or alcohol. The third category is one that most people have trouble understanding and that involves emotional components like anxiety, stress or depression.

Although there are many different initial reasons we may start having back pain it will usually start off as a muscular injury. Most of us are familiar with this type of condition. We have all pulled a muscle at one time or another. An injured muscle will tighten and develop painful knots points. It does this to help protect the injury. Think of a rope that you need to shorten in order to maintain tension, one way to do this is place a big knot in the rope. These knots are known as trigger points because they are sore to touch and trigger pain. They are small places in the muscle where there is not enough blood circulating which gives an opportunity for chemicals that cause pain to build up. If the muscle is not properly lengthened it will start pulling your spinal joints out of alignment and cause nerve irritation.

A misaligned joint is called a spinal subluxation. This places stress on your ligaments and nerves which causes pain and prevents full range of motion.Eventually the torque caused by incorrect movement of your joints will damage your discs. These cushions serve as shock absorbers between the bones and maintain room for the nerves. A disc bulges or disc herniation can compress the spinal nerve causing severe pain that will eventually led to numbness and loss of function. The most common symptom of a damaged disc is sciatica, or pain that travels into the buttocks and down the leg.

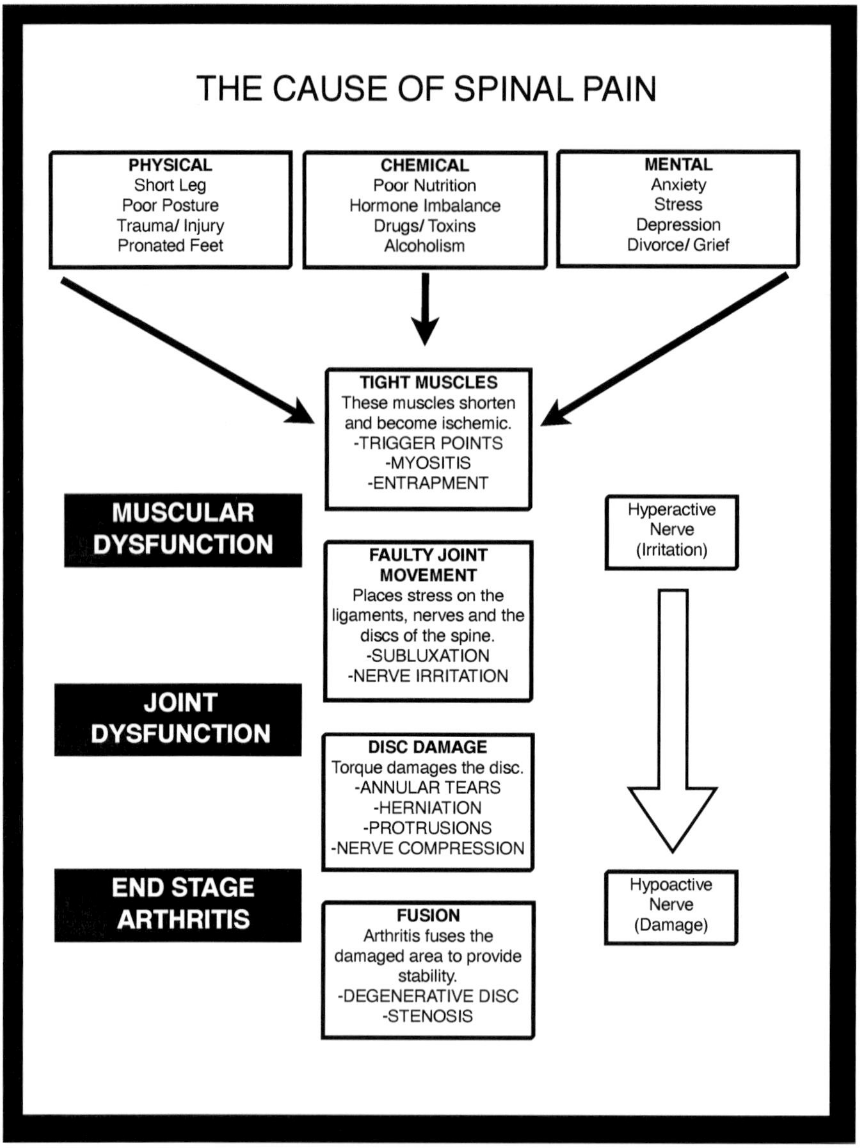

When left untreated a damaged disc starts to degenerate. This is commonly known as degenerative disc disease or DDD for short. This is your body's way of trying to stabilize the injury and prevent further damage. In extreme cases spinal stenosis occurs. Stenosis is what happens when arthritis fills in the nerve openings in your spine. This causes leg pain and inability to walk very far. Until recently the only solution for stenosis was considered to be back surgery.

The entire process is degenerative in nature and the further along it gets the harder it is to reverse. In the beginning nerves get over excited or hyperactive and as they are exposed to continuous irritation they slow down and become hypoactive, eventually leading to loss of function.

This illustrates why it is so important to always treat injuries as soon as they occur. Spending a little time working on trigger points you developed while on the computer will prevent arthritis down the road. The body is not unlike a machine and it needs to be maintained. Many times a person is not even aware that they have trigger points or subluxations until the damage is already done.

The Examination

I have developed a systematic way of evaluating a patient regardless of their complaint. I call this my 10 Point Examination. This is a standard of care that leaves no stone unturned in determining the true cause of the patients condition. Some of these tests are more medical based, things like getting blood and urine samples and not normally part of a chiropractor's bag of clinical tools. I realized early on that if I wanted to see the whole picture I would need to use whatever means were available to me. One blessing to my clinical practice has been using a state certified medical assistant to help with many of these tasks. Carol Bailey Niemela MA, RCA, is certainly one of the best. She can draw blood, inject B12 or assist in more invasive medical procedures whenever they are necessary (under the supervision of a medical doctor). Carole has worked with a Stanford neurosurgeon and a board certified anesthesiologist. She is highly skilled technically but perhaps, even more important, Carol has a bedside manner that would put even the most seasoned nurse to shame. Patients absolutely love her and she can really deliver in tough cases that require focus and thinking out of the box. She is a perfect combination of traditional medicine with a holistic intent.

Here is a summary of my 10 point examination I preform on all my patients regardless of the complaint.

1. Comprehensive History

A complete review of your health history and list of all injuries and sicknesses. Sometimes there is trauma in the past that patients may have overlooked as insignificant but later we discover it was the initial start of their problem. In a few cases I have found injury that occurred during the birthing process to be a contributing factor to a patients current problem. Every injury you have experienced will be recorded in your cellular memory. We have to create a map of why your body has stopped healing. This takes the most time, is the most important part of the exam and ironically is the most lacking in most patient doctor encounters. Sometimes this will take 30 minutes, other times it may take an hour. In rare cases, I will split the history over several visits if necessary but I make sure I get all the information regardless of the time needed. I also like to use functional evaluation forms like the Oswestry questionnaire which will give the patient an overall disability rating based on what they can and cannot do during their normal lives. For most patients it is not pain but loss of function that they are most upset about.

2. Structural X-Rays

Medical x-rays are usually done lying down and therefore do not show the effects of gravity. I always take x-rays standing up. In this position I can see how things like short legs, joint alignment, scoliosis and degeneration affect the body. Many times we find things overlooked in basic medical x-rays done at an imaging center. In some case, I will also take x-rays while moving the patient in various positions. For example, I frequently find a condition called Spondylolisthesis when x-raying a patient bending forward and then backward. The vertebra will slip and compress the spinal cord. This type of unusual x-ray will reveal hidden problems. Another favorite of my lateral side bending because it will show coupled motion pathology of the spinal joints.

3. Nervoscope Evaluation

Only a chiropractor is licensed to check your spine for subluxations and the nervoscope evaluation is a traditional tool to help in that process. It compares temperature on either side of your spine. A sudden increase in temperature usually means there is inflammation present and irritation to the spinal nerve. This is a fast and simple test that most chiropractors have stopped doing because medical doctors reject it. But they just don't understand the science. I document before and after scans on my patients and I see remarkable changes as they improve or little change is they do not. The greatest benefit of the nervoscope is the ability to identify areas of the spine where problems exist despite the lack of symptoms. Since only about 10% of your nerves are sensory pain is not a reliable indicator. The nervoscope is one of my most powerful tools for finding subacute problems.

I have a local neurologist who gets regular adjustments from me and he insists that I use my nervoscope before and after I adjust him. Honestly, I think he is considering buying this device for his own practice. The nervoscope I use is made by Tytronics. I encourage anyone interested in the science behind thermography to contact them. Currently Tytronics is using this technology as a non invasive method to screen for breast cancer. Remarkable equipment that my patients are fortunate to benefit from.

4. Neurological Testing

Testing all the main nerves of the body and seeing how the brain reacts when I stimulate them is a standard in my exams. The most important nerves are the 12 cranial. These come directly off the brain and represent a window into the patient's health. I also evaluate the Cerebellum, do blind spot mapping and check deep tendon reflexes. I want to know how the body responds to vibration, a pin prick, to heat and cold. These tests are not expensive to preform so patients can be retested frequently. I will often test before and after a single treatment to asses the effectiveness of a particular modality. When someone cannot feel vibration in their big toe and then after removing a subluxation or using laser on their nerve root there's a response, well that's powerful.

5. Muscle Testing

Muscle dysfunction can damage joints and irritate nerves. I learned all about muscles from my time spent with Dr. Fiscella. It is important to always test the main muscles of the body for proper function. The same nerves that control these muscles also innervate the organs of the body. Here is an example,

The Tibialis Anterior, a muscle on the front of your lower leg, is neurologically linked to your urinary bladder. So problem with the bladder can present as dysfunction of this muscle and visa-versa.

Muscle testing is of vital importance yet the medical community has forgotten the vital connection between muscles and organs. I frequently will uncover potential health problems before they arise by testing the major muscles of the body. In one patient they had a very weak Tensor Fascia Lata muscle which is related to the large intestine. Although they had no symptoms, I decided to run some further tests on the colon and discovered several problems that were easily corrected. If untreated this hidden condition may have developed into cancer.

6. Palpation

This is really a lost art. Checking the joints and organs of the body for correct motion and tone is called palpation. Many times a skilled doctor will tell you what is wrong simply by touch. I can check the position of the liver, spleen and kidneys and if there are restrictions I can also manipulate them into correct motion. The best example of this is a Hiatal hernia. I must have fixed

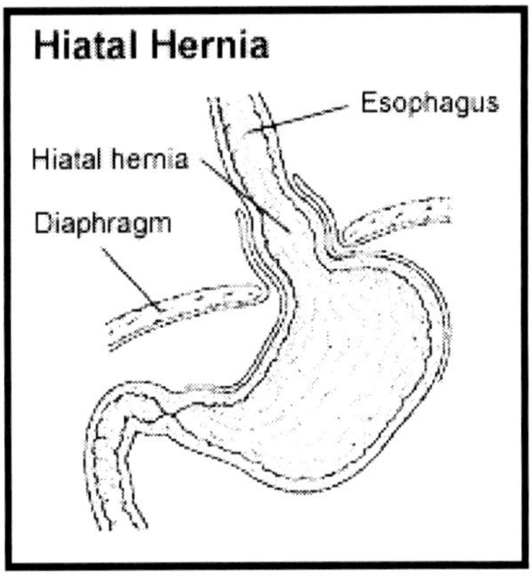

hundreds of these over the years by pulling the stomach down out of the throat. People are amazed that this stuff is possible without surgery. This hands on approach is becoming quickly replaced with drugs and invasive procedures. A few years ago my father in-law, John Park, had a large inguinal hernia and was in severe pain. With the help of Dr. Paul Arnold, a very skilled osteopath in his own right, we pushed the colon back into place and instantly relieved all his pain. It is such a shame that more physicians don't take the time to develop these skills. A word of thanks to the good Dr. Arnold. The last time I checked Dr. Arnold was still running an osteopathic practice in Cape Coral, Florida.

7. Health Vitals

Bilateral blood pressure, oxygen levels, pulse, body temperature, height and weight can help diagnose underlying conditions.

•Temperature: 98.6' F
•Pulse Rate: 72 bpm men, 80 bpm women
•Respiratory Rate: 8-16 cpm
•Blood Pressure: 110 to 140/ 60 to 90 mm Hg
•Height to Weight Ratio
•Chest Expansion: 2-4 inches
•Blood Oxygen Saturation Level: 100%

Vitals are done every visit. When was the last time your physician took your blood pressure 3 times to get an accurate number and did both sides of your body? You need to compare your right side to the left side for a complete picture. How about checking the difference in your blood pressure when you move from a sitting position to standing? Do you know what your blood oxygen saturation index is? My patients are taught how to self monitor these numbers with home care equipment and what is considered normal.

8. Urine Evaluation

Every patient receives a Urinalysis (UA) in the office as part of the 10 Point Examination. This gives a foundation from which I can start creating their metabolic profile. Many hidden or subacute health problems are uncovered from this test. Even a few years ago UA's were expensive and hard to preform but today anyone can buy these urine test strips from a local drug store or on the internet. I have convinced many of my patients to test their urine at home. This way they can monitor their health and the effectiveness of things like dietary or supplementation programs.

Here is a breakdown of the most important elements to the urine study, as you will see there is a large amount of information available from an inexpensive test,

•Specific Gravity

Measures the ability to concentrate and excrete your in the kidneys. Less than 1.015 indicates either high intake of water, very low electrolytes, decreased kidney function, or diabetes. More than 1.015 indicates dehydration, diabetes, decreased kidney function, congestive heart failure, liver failure, shock.

•pH

Normal pH is between 6.0 to 6.8. A pH between 5.0 and 6.0 indicates an acidic environment this could be due to high protein diet with mineral buffer deficiency, digestion or torsion problems, acidosis or fever. When the pH of the urine is between 7.0 and 9.0 this indicates an alkaline environment and can be the result of a vegetarian diet, urinary tract infections, metabolic or respiratory alkalosis. But, it is usually an indication of infection. Remember your body maintains it's pH naturally, this test indicates how much stress it is under to do that job.

•Leukocytes

There shouldn't be any leukocytes in your urine, these are white blood cells and always indicate the presence of inflammation and infection.

•Nitrates

Nitrates are not normally present in the urine. The presence of urinary nitrate may indicate bacterial contamination or infection in the bladder. Usually this indicates a UTI.

•Protein

Normally protein, because of its molecular size, is not excreted in the urine. Trace amounts can show up due to severe muscular strain, emotional stress, pregnancy, fever, trauma and ingestion of hard water. More significant amounts indicate kidney disease.

•Glucose

Glucose should not be detected in normal urine and can indicates diabetes, kidney stress or Cushing's syndrome. This is a common finding although not normal.

•Ketones

When your body uses fatty acids as fuel it produces ketones. If I'm doing a supervised fast with the patient I expect to see ketones in the urine by the third day. This would indicate the body has switched over to burning fat as fuel instead of glucose. If the patient is not fasting then the presence of ketones in the urine is an indication of diabetic ketosis, and needs to be further examined. Ketone strips are now available in any drug store and popular with the popular Atkin's style protein diet.

•Urobilinogen

Liver damage, hepatitis, hemolytic disorders, biliary obstruction, and severe infection are all possibilities when this is positive.

•Bilirubin

This an indication of inflammation of the liver and biliary stasis or the presence of gallstones impeding the flow of bile into the small intestine. I see it in cases of hepatitis, cirrhosis, liver disease, and bile obstruction. Also this can be present if the patient is taking drugs that are toxic to the liver. Usually I will look for jaundice in these cases.

•Blood

Unless the patient is a menstruating female there should be no blood in the urine. There will be two types noted on your test strip. Non-hemolyzed can mean UTI, glomerular nephritis or strenuous exercise. Hemolyzed may be the result of allergies, or liver inflammation.

9. Blood Work

In some cases of Chronic Pain, blood lab work is needed. I am not qualified to draw blood out of a patient's arm and trust me, it is not something you would want me to do. Luckily I have several medical assistants that are very good at it and while I don't do the draw, I am fully educated in clinical interpretation of the results. The most important tests for my average patient are:

•Thyroid Panel (thyroid antibodies: TPO-Ab and TBG)
•Complete Metabolic Panel (CMP)
•Lipid Panel
•CBC (complete blood chemistry)
•Food Sensitivity Testing
•Adrenal Stress Index
•Immune Panels
•H. Pylori
•Intestinal Permeability
•Homocysteine levels and C-Reactive Protein

I also like to look at the blood in real time. This is done using a phase contrast microscope and a small finger stick sample placed on a slide. Live cell analysis allows a doctor to get a big picture view of what is happening in real time. For me there is no better motivator for a sick patient than showing them their live blood on a TV screen. Imagine watching as a white blood cell eats a piece of invading bacteria. I have people coming to my clinic just for this one test. It only takes about 30 minutes and the patient gets to see a world they never before knew existed. It is most useful when I want to show a patient a before and after picture of how a diet, supplements or even stress has affected their health. The most common findings relate to faulty digestion and transportation of oxygen, usually the red blood cells are all clumped together. This is one of the first things that will change as health improves.

10. Documentation

The 10th point in the examination is patient education. It is important that the patient understands what is wrong with them and how they can help improve the condition. You cannot fight your demons unless you name them so I give every patient a complete, typed report of all exam findings and recommendations for care. Printed on quality paper, indexed and signed by myself and all people who were involved in the examination process. Then I go over everything with them step by step, line by line. It is usually about 8 pages long. I refuse to cut corners or duplicate previous conclusions without proper testing because more than 30% of the time I will find errors. That's a big deal when you are taking about someones health, especially when it is your health. The report is more like a roadmap that shows the patient where they have been and where they need to go. This book grew out of the process of creating this patient report of findings. Most patients need at least some help in each of the 7 steps to innate healing that are covered in this book.

Red Flags

I am very much in favor of self treatment however there are certain circumstances where yo need to see your doctor. These are known as red flags. Anytime a patient has any of these it is important to seek professional help. Even in my clinic there are occasions where I will refer patients out for medical care. Any patient experiencing the following symptoms should consult with a physician immediately.

•Pain is severe or worsens when lying down
•Fever over 100' Fahrenheit
•Pain is present for over a month
•Unexplained weight loss
•History of cancer
•History of long term steroid use
•Recent inset of urinary tract problems
•Pain is related to a trauma
•Severe weakness or numbness
•Problems with urinating or having a bowel movement

What To Start Doing Right Now

The following are excellent suggestions for any patient in pain and reflect my functional medicine training. These supplements are inexpensive and available everywhere. The first two products will make you feel better, the next three reduce inflammation, which is a primary cause of pain, the next three speed up tissue healing and the final one supports the emotional component of your condition. Of course I do not recommend that you take all these together, instead find the right combination that works for you. If one product makes you feel funny or upsets your stomach stop taking it and try another one in it's category. Some patients take 2 or 3 products others need most of them. Every case is different. Remember you are not my patient and these are only guidelines, please read the disclaimer at the front of the book and use common sense when considering undertaking any form of self treatment. If something is powerful enough to heal it is also strong enough to harm will also harm.

There are trivial truths and the great truths. The opposite of a trivial truth is plainly false. The opposite of a great truth is also true. -Niels Bohr

To Relieve Pain

Reducing pain is different from repairing damaged tissue. This is something many people and most doctors seem to forget. Pain is a symptom that something is wrong. Feeling better is important but always dig deeper to correct the cause of your pain. These products help your body use chemicals that make you feel better. Long term they are not a solution because they do not target the underlying issues but short term they can give you a much needed break from pain without the dangerous side effects of prescription medication.

1. DL-phenylalanine: 1000-4000 mg twice a day on an empty stomach.

DL-phenylalanine (DLPA) will make you feel better by reducing pain. This was the first product I started giving patients when I got my biochemical wall charts from Roche because I could see how DLPA inhibited endorphin degradation leading to an inhibition of GABA release in the midbrain to cause greater dopamine production. This produces an antidepressant effect. Endorphins are more powerful than morphine and your body makes them naturally. One of the biggest problems with patient's taking a narcotic prescription pain killer like OxyContin is that it reduces your body's ability to produce endorphins. I have seen DLPA help patients as they get off these dangerous narcotics but it can elevate blood pressure and cause rapid heart beat so you need to start with the lowest dose that produces a desirable level of relief.

WARNING: You cannot use DLPA or L-tyrosine if you are taking MAO or tricyclic anti depressants.

2. White Willow Bark (Salizan) - 1000 mg every 4 hours

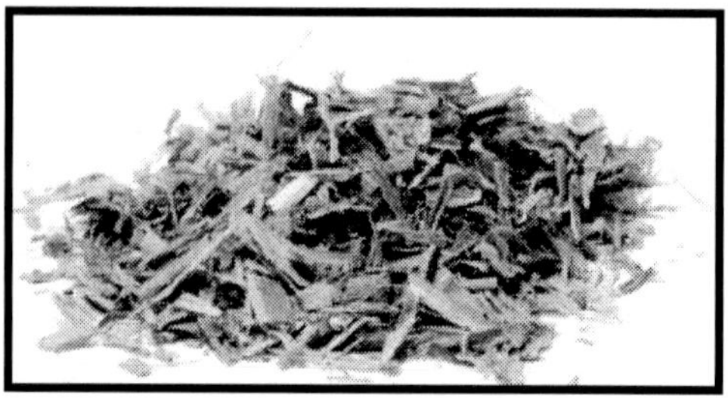

Salizain is concentrated white willow bark, which has been used for centuries as a natural remedy for aches and pains. Research has demonstrated that pain relief from white willow is similar to prescription anti-inflammatory drugs. The American College of Physicians and the American Pain Society developed clinical guidelines for the treatment of low back pain, which included the use of white willow bark Each tablet contains almost 1000 mg of white willow bark, which provides 240 mg of salicin per tablet. This natural component is similar to the active ingredient found in aspirin. White willow also contains anti-inflammatory and analgesic tannins, flavonoids, and polyphenols. Side effects are similar to placebos, which makes white willow a safe alternative to anti-inflammatory drugs for pain relief. Anabolic Labs is the best resource for white willow bark and salicin. Patients can take a few thousand mgs. as needed every 4-6 hours.

WARNING: You cannot use White Willow Bark if you are sensitive to Asprin.

3. Cryroderm - Every 2 - 3 hours

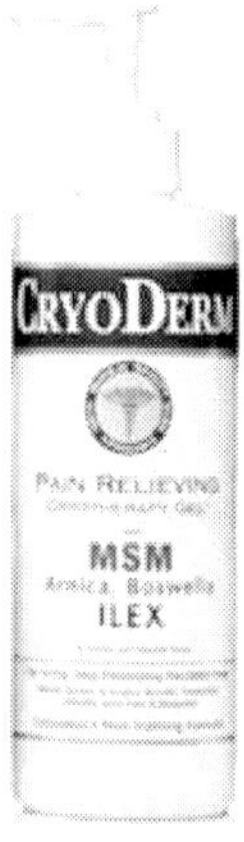

This is an amazing product that will help your body recover from injury by helping it regain balance, known in the medical field as homeostasis. It contains a high level of Menthol, which will immediately reduce pain but the mechanism of how this product works provides for much more benefit. When your muscles or joints are inflamed, such as after trauma, exertion, or in arthritis, the blood vessels become leaky and let plasma, white blood cells, and

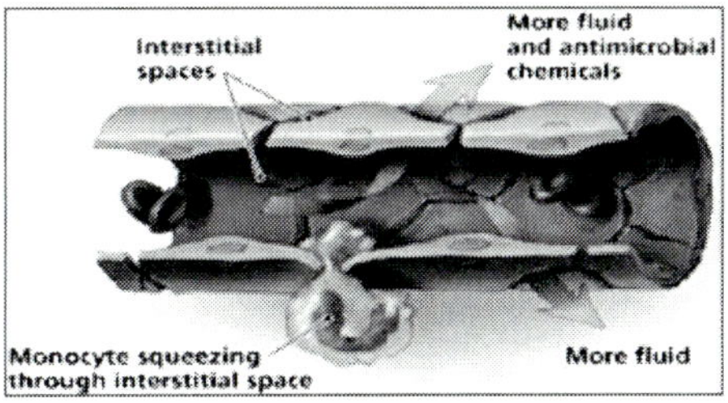

cytokines-the so-called "inflammatory soup" out into the surrounding tissue. The tissue becomes red, warm, swollen, and painful. CRYODERM'S® proprietary formulation counteracts the vasodilatory effects of the inflammatory mediators making blood vessels contract. This reduces swelling, redness, inflammation, eliminates pain, discomfort and restores the tissue homeostasis.

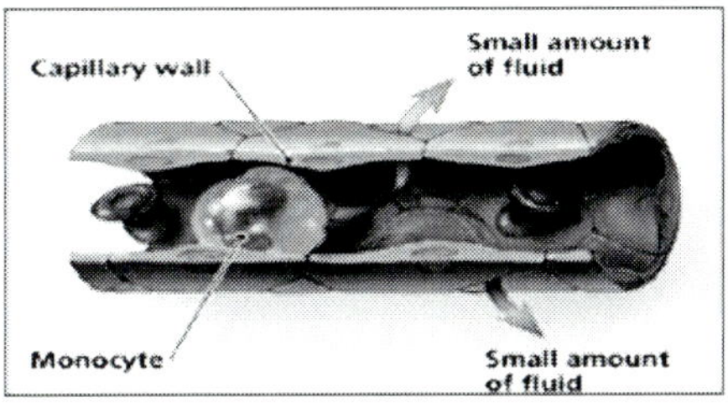

When your muscles are in spasm, the blood vessels are constricted, reducing the blood flow to the area and depriving the tissue of the vital oxygen. In this scenario CRYODERM'S® proprietary formulation causes relaxation of blood vessels and a reduction in sympathetic nerve-mediated contraction. CRYODERM® helps restore the natural balance by dilating the blood vessels, thus improving microcirculation, tissue oxygen supply, removing the toxic by-products of metabolism, resolving interstitial acidosis and speeding up tissue healing. So CRYODERM® aids in regulating blood flow depending on the tissue state, restoring natural homeostasis.

The product is free of dangerous chemicals and can be used repeatedly throughout the day. There are other products on the market that may seem the same but in my clinical trials only CRYODERM® can produce such safe long lasting effects.

To Reduce Inflammation

Inflammation is a protective step taken to initiate the healing process. Without inflammation, wounds and infections would never heal. Similarly, progressive destruction of the tissue would compromise the survival of the organism. However, chronic inflammation can also lead to a host of diseases, such as hay fever, periodontitis, atherosclerosis, rheumatoid arthritis, and even cancer (e.g., gallbladder carcinoma). It is for that reason that inflammation needs to be closely regulated by the body. It is important in the healing process but in chronic conditions it can get out of control, prevent repair and cause disease.

1. Harpagophytum Procumbens (Devils Claw): 600 - 1,200 mg, standardized to contain 50 - 100 mg of harpagoside, 3 times daily.

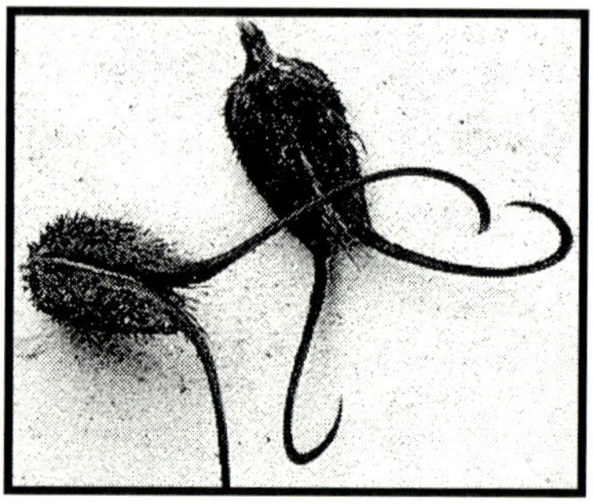

Devil's claw is an herb. The botanical name, Harpagophytum, means "hook plant" in Greek. This plant, which is native to Africa, gets its name from the appearance of its fruit, which is covered with hooks meant to attach onto animals in order to spread the seeds. This is not the same as Cat's Claw, there is a big difference, so please pay attention and get the right stuff. Imagine a product that is as good as Vioxx but without all the side effects that forced Vioxx off the market. That's Devils Claw. A great COX-2 inhibitor that can reduce your pain, especially good for arthritic, degenerative pain seen mostly in the elderly or in low back cases. Devils Claw not only makes you feel better but it changes how your central nervous system responds to pain. A great product that I prescribe daily to all my arthritic patients. It's primary purpose is pain reduction. Many times I use Devils Claw as a front line product especially when there is not much inflammation present and I just want them to get a break from all the pain receptor activity. In my own personal struggle with chronic pain, Devils Claw was my most effective supplement. Like every product in this book you will need to test results for yourself, but for me Devils Claw was a big part of my relief.

2. Zinger Officinale (GINGER): 1000-4000 mg a day, standardized 5% Gingerols and Shogaols extract

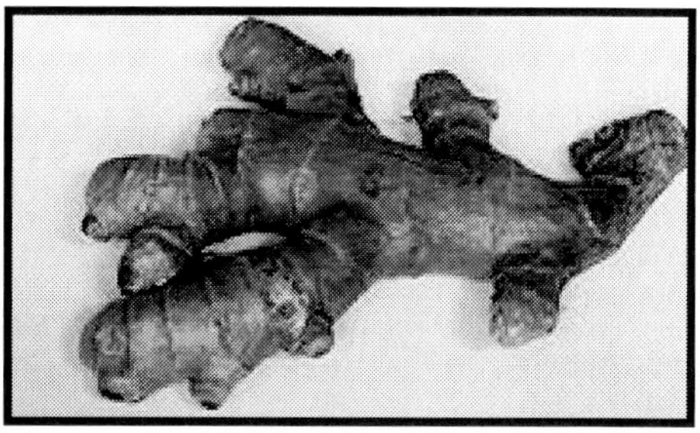

Ginger has been around for over 3,000 years, the effectiveness of this herb comes from the dried roots oils known as gingerols and shogaols. This herb reduces Prostaglandins but also formation of Substance P. So it is a great herb to take as a preventive measure. Start by ramping up your dosage until you find a level that gives you the desired relief but after about 6 weeks you should be able to lower your intake to a maintenance level, (500-1000 mg a day works good). I recommend taking with food and dividing up your daily dose equally. Recently ginger has been found to produce a chemotherapeutic effects on colon cancer. As if there is not already enough reasons to take ginger! You cannot just eat ginger root in your Chinese stir fry because the heat will destroy the useful elements.

3. Turmeric: 1000-3000 mg a day, standardized 95% Curcuminoids extract

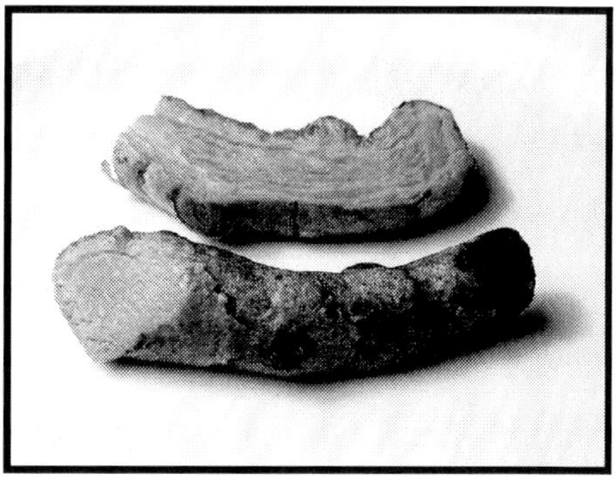

Turmeric has been around for over 5,000 years! It comes from the Curcumin Longa root and is found primarily in Southern India, think curry dishes. It is the most powerful anti-inflammation product available. This is the magic bullet. Results surpass NSAIDS and Hydrocortisone without the dangerous side effects. There are currently over 1500 valid, scientific research papers proving the wonderful effects of turmeric on pain and inflammation (just google). Turmeric is special because it inhibits activation of something called NF-Kappa B, a pain producing chemical. You need to be certain you are getting a standardized 95% product when you buy turmeric. Hydrocarbons are the nasty things that are made when we burn things, think BBQ, smoking, air pollution from our cars or burnt toast. Hydrocarbons cause cancer and turmeric prevents the formation of these cancers. In case you missed what I just said, turmeric prevents cancer.

One company that I have always used to buy many of the herbs I use in clinic is Tattva's Herbs. They are "the" source for Turmeric and Ginger. Below is an explanation of their manufacturing process,

There is simply no other extraction method so effective that you can smell the purity, fragrance and essence of the herb. This is a testimony to the great care that goes into the selection of the herbs and the supercritical extraction process itself. To give you an idea of the potency and concentration of the extract, we can often use as much as 200 to 250 pounds of fresh herbs to produce just one pound of supercritical extract.

All of the herbs are grown on organic farms and selected with the greatest of care. The supercritical process produces an exceptionally broad representation of the herbs' active constituents, which often times traditional methods of extraction cannot even begin to extract. Furthermore, the supercritical process does not use any chemical solvents at all. Instead, it utilizes safe and environmentally friendly carbon dioxide, the same carbon dioxide that is found in your sparkling water.

Finally, the supercritical extract, post-supercritical extract (PSE) (a water-soluble extract), and the raw whole herb are combined to create our herbal formulas. The finished product is superior in terms of both freshness and breadth of active constituents. It delivers the full spectrum of the herbs with a potency that cannot be surpassed. In addition, all the herbs are independently tested for heavy metals and other contaminates. The result is an exquisite formula that delivers simplicity, purity and incredible potency all at once.

The finished product is superior in terms of both freshness and breadth of active constituents. It delivers the full spectrum of the herbs with a potency that cannot be surpassed. In addition, all of the herbs are independently tested for heavy metals and other contaminates. The result is an exquisite formula that delivers simplicity, purity and incredible potency all at once.

4. EPA/DHA (Omega 3 Fatty Acids): 3,000-5,000 mg day

In my clinic this is known as doing an oil change. One of the best ways to manage systemic inflammation is by taking an omega 3 fatty acids supplement. Studies have shown that specific fatty acids, known as EPA and DHA lowers inflammation in human tissue. This was first discovered when the Inuit people, who had diets high in animal fats, had low incidence of heart disease, inflammatory bowel disease, asthma and psoriasis.

These oils are naturally anti-inflammatory because they inhibit the conversion of arachidonic acid to pro-inflammatory chemicals (prostaglandin E2, thromboxane A2 and leukotriene B4, as well as the pro-inflammatory cytokines, tumor necrosis factor alpha (TNF-a) and interleukin 1 alpha). Omega 3 also significantly prevents the conversion of arachidonic acid to the enzyme cyclo-oxygenase COX-2. Drugs like Celebrex operate on this COX-2 pathway.

If you find that taking an NSAID (non steroidal anti-inflammatory drug) like Advil or Aleve reduces your pain then that is a positive test you already have an omega 3 fatty acid deficiency. NSAIDS won't work unless the deficiency is present. So whenever someone tells me that NSAIDS help, I immediately get them on high dosages of fatty acids and they usually will start feeling improvement within 48 hours.

You will needed very high dosages of EPA and most fish oil capsules will not be able to supply enough active product. Look at the back of the bottle and see how much EPA is in the capsule, you maybe shocked to find out that your 1000 mg fish oil capsule only contains 200 mg of EPA. Remember you need 3,000-5,000 mg of EPA. One fish oil product I have found to be effective is made by Barlens. A single teaspoon has 850 mg of EPA, so you can easily get up to several thousand milligrams a day.

There is one exception for those who want capsules and that is Arctic Fresh fish oil capsules. This was formulated by Dr. David Edmund Ruggieri, MD of, Center for Health, Punta Gorda, Florida. www.articfresh.com

Dr. Ruggieri's speciality is cardiovascular disease and he created his own fish oil product to help his patients. Just 2 capsules contains 1152 mg EPA. This is an impressive amount of EPA. I recommend this product and the good doctor to anyone interested in reversing or preventing heart disease.

There is some confusion about omega 3 oils that I want to clear up. Some doctors tell patients to take flax seed oil in instead of fish oils because the body has enzymes that can convert alpha linolenic acid (ALA) omega fatty acids into EPA/DHA. This is true however it is impossible to convert enough to achieve the high levels needed to lower inflammation of a sick patient. Many chronically sick patients have a defect in their biochemistry so they are unable to convert the omega 3's into EPA/DHA so the flax seed oil is mostly ineffective. I highly recommend fish oil over flax. The fish oil has many more benefits to your health besides lowering inflammation. It really has a "big wow" factor that patients see and feel very quickly and this includes dramatic changes to dangerously high blood lab levels.

Never start taking fish oil if you are already on medications for cardiovascular health without consulting your doctor. This is especially important if you are taking blood thinners.

To Assist Healing

Okay, so we have just covered the essential products you take to feel better. They will reduce or block the chemicals that are causing your pain and that's a good thing, no doubt, but there are some other incredible supplements you need to consider that work on helping the cells heal. These do not directly reduce pain, but they promote cellular growth. They are just as important and I find that in older patients (anyone over 40) they really are essential.

1. Amino Acids: Take an essential Amino Acid supplement.

There are some 22 Amino Acids but there are only 8 that are known as essential (some argue 10). These are necessary to make the rest and you need to make sure you are getting all of them in your diet. Specifically the essential amino acids are,

•valine
•leucine
•isoleucine
•phenylalanine
•threonine
•methionine
•lysine
•tryptophan

Some research indicates that these two are also essential,
•histidine
•cystine

If you have these 8 (10) essential amino acids you can make the others from the foods you eat. It's these essential amino acids which are most likely to be deficient in the diet because although they are found in animal products such as eggs and meat, they are quickly destroyed by heat. So maybe a person is eating lots of meat but if it is over cooked the nutritional value is low. In this case the amino acids are not used by the cells and instead just circulate in the blood stream. So when a person starts taking an amino acid supplement I first see the protein in the blood start to go down because the amino acids are starting to be used by the cells. The main symptom indicating a need for essential amino acids supplementation is fatigue. Amino acids are also responsible for making neurotransmitters (brain mood chemicals) which we cover later in step 7.

There are many good products on the market, personally I find many bodybuilding/ weightlifting gyms are great sources for amino supplementation. It is hard to justify a 100% vegetarian diet when we know these 8 (10) essential amino acids come directly from animal products. We will discuss this more in step 5. It was a direct result of my studying of amino acids and neurotransmitter therapy that I began to question the long term implications of a vegetarian diet.

2. RNA (Ribonucleic Acid): 0.5 to 1.5 grams daily.

Ribonucleic Acid is usually called RNA. It's role in cell multiplication and development is huge. RNA helps build cells by supporting protein synthesis. In the body, RNA helps to transfer genetic messages from the DNA to guide the manufacture of proteins using the amino acids that are extracted from foods or created by the body. What this means in practical terms for medicine is that the RNA can direct the synthesis of proteins. This is an amazingly powerful role. It doesn't matter if the proteins you are talking about are proteins involved in heart disease, cholesterol metabolism, or weight management, RNA can help the body heal. If protein isn't being used at the cellular level, it's likely to be present in the blood and this can block circulation and cause problems such as cold hands and feet. Clinically, these patients improve once you give them RNA. We also know that formation of white blood cells is inhibited by a deficiency of nucleic acid, so RNA supplementation can be helpful to people with immune compromise. Whenever you are trying to heal tissue I like to increase amino acid intake and then use RNA as the director to make sure the job gets done. There is a Dr. Frank of New York City who wrote a book ribonucleic acid. He knew that if amino acids could not be used by the cells they would circulate in the blood and cause coldness and circulating problems in the extremities. Dr. Frank gave his patients high doses of RNA and the condition cleared up. With the RNA we can help drive amino acids to where they can be used. One source that you can make this from is yeast extract. There are many suppliers of RNA available and it is not expensive, I personally like Standard Process.

3. Gotu Kola (Centella Asiatica): 1000 mg Day

Gotu Kola has been used to treat a number of conditions for thousands of years in India, China, and Indonesia. It has been called "the fountain of life" because legend has it that an ancient Chinese herbalist lived for more than 200 years as a result of taking Gotu Kola. Historically, Gotu Kola has also been used to treat syphilis, hepatitis, stomach ulcers, mental fatigue, epilepsy, diarrhea, fever, and asthma.

Angiogenesis is the ability for the body to grow new blood vessels and it is a necessary part of the healing process. Gotu Kola primarily increases this activity and therefore is useful in any condition that needs to promote tissue healing. Diabetic neuropathy, ulcers, burns, cellulitis, scleroderma and most importantly damaged muscles, ligaments and spinal discs all can benefit from Gotu Kola. In chronic, inflammatory conditions Gotu Kola is the best resource to prevent fibrosis formation. Since it also increase blood flow to the brain it can be helpful in prevention of disorders like dementia. The herb smells awful but works quickly. Please note that Gotu Kola is not the same as Kola Nut (Cola Nitida) which is a stimulant. You do not want to use this product if you are battling cancer because angiogenesis can cause cancer to spread by growing new blood vessels into the mutated cells, giving them strength.

Emotional Support

There is no denying that all pain has an emotional component. If we look at where the emotional centers of the brain are located we see they are close to the areas that register nociception. So emotions have a direct influence on how sensitive we are to pain. Anyone interested in learning more about this relationship should read the research of Dr. John Sarno, MD.

Mind Over Back Pain: A radically New Approach To The Diagnosis And Treatment Of Back Pain

Dr. Sarno was the Professor of Clinical Rehabilitation Medicine at New York University School of Medicine and attending physician at the Howard A Rusk Institute of Rehabilitation Medicine New York University Medical Center. He makes a very good case for his Tension Myositis Syndrome (TMS) as a primary cause of chronic pain. I use many of his techniques in treating my own patients with excellent results. I even produced a DVD lecture that summarizes Dr. Sarno's work on TMS that I give to all my new chronic pain patients as required viewing.

I am not a psychologist, but I recognize the need to reduce anxiety and stress in patients trying to initiate the innate healing response. St. John's Wort is very effective in filling this role and it is a real help to patients that are depressed or suffering from anxiety. I see patients improve in both mood and over all well being. One of the most outstanding properties of St. John's Wort and one that is never advertised is it's antiviral activity. It is very unique and I will prescribe it for viral infections like herpes, Epstein Barr virus, and other enveloped viral infections. It will not work on non-enveloped viruses such as human papaloma virus, which causes warts. Most of the hepatitis viruses are enveloped except for hepatitis A. Start with a few thousand milligrams per day and adjust accordingly.

1. St. John's Wort: 2000-3000 mg Day

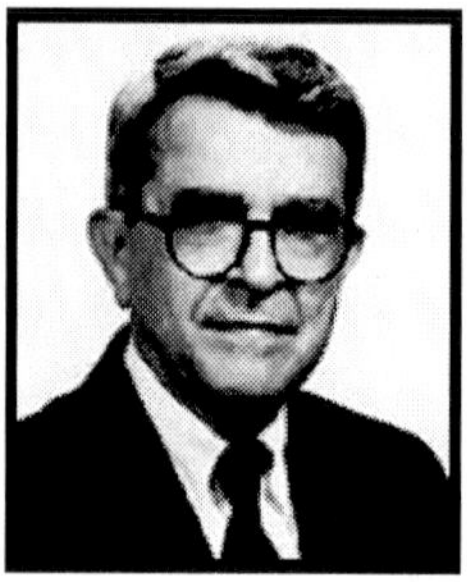

I have a theory that chronic pain syndromes, including back pain, have a viral component. At this time, I am still collecting data but my personal research seems to be indicating that many if not all chronic problems are viral in nature. Of course the implication here is that you could literally catch back pain from someone else. Clinically, I have seen this on many occasions and my observations suggests that a viral component attacks the immune system and increases the body's sensitivity to pain. Of course there are many other pieces to this puzzle but for now, I believe that St. John's Wort is a very good idea. There are critics but most negative results have to do with not using a standardized extract. The only supplier of St. John's Wort that I have found to produce a reliable extract is Mediherb. In addition to emotional support I prescribe it frequently in combination with immune enhancing herbs for viral infections such as herpes, Epstein-Barr virus and other envelope viral infections. It will not work on non-enveloped viruses like human papaloma virus, which causes warts. Most of the hepatitis viruses are envelope the exception of hepatitis A which is non-envelope.

Medical Magnets

I want the general public to know that science isn't run the way they read about it in the newspapers and magazines. I want lay people to understand that they cannot automatically accept scientists' pronouncements at face value, for too often they're self-serving and misleading. I want our citizens, nonscientists as well as investigators to work to change the way research is administered. The way it's currently funded and evaluated, we're learning more and more about less and less, and science is becoming our enemy instead of our friend.
- Dr. Robert O. Becker, MD

Dr. Becker wrote two famous books about magnetic fields and the implications for healing and damaging the human body. I do not understand how these cannot be essential part of any medical curriculum. They should be part of your personal health collection. The books are,

The Body Electric: Electromagnetism The Foundation of Life

Cross Currents: The Perils of Electropollution, The Promise of Electromedicine.

You will never look at your cell phone or electric razor the same again. Many years ago, I was working in a large clinic and I had this one patient that I just could not get better. After trying everything, I went to my senior supervisor and pleaded for some help. The doctor went into the examination room and palpated the patient,

We are going to have to use some advanced medicine on his patient Dr. Stokes.

The Doctor reached into his bag and took out two rectangular objects, approximately 8" x 3" and about half an inch thick. I had no idea what was about to happen. He paused for a moment studying the markings on these two objects, then finally announced,

The patient is suffering from inflammation and his energy field is out of sync, today we will use the north pole.

He placed the two objects, north side down, against the patient's lower back and that was it. What? Come on I thought, you have to be kidding? Energy fields, magnets, this was too much. I started rehearsing how I was going to apologize to my patients for this display of nonsense. The older doctor continued,

Today we will only do 10 minutes, once he starts feeling better we must switch the magnets to the south pole to stimulate tissue growth. The north pole is for inflammation Dr. Stokes or to slow down energy production, the south pole is for growth or to speed up the energy.

What could I do? I was the young associate, he was the experienced physician. This was all coming from the same doctor that just a few hours before I had seen diagnose Chondromyxoid Fibroma on a 25 years old patients tibia (a very rare bone tumor that represents less than 1% of all bone neoplasms). So I nodded my head and agreed, north pole, south pole, Santa Claus, Easter bunny, got it. The next day my patient was 50% improved. I was prepared to apologize for the magnet treatment but instead found myself repeating the procedure at the patients request. The magnets, he stated, worked great! After more study, I discovered a huge amount of evidence-based research that proved beyond any doubt that magnetic fields have direct influence upon cellular healing and our health.

The Earth is a giant magnet with a North and a South Pole. A few hundred years ago the magnetic field of the earth registered in the strength of 4 gauss. Today it is about 1/2 a gauss. A human being produces a magnetic field of only 1 gauss, which means that as we live and walk around we are being drained. There is now a tremendous amount of evidence proving electromagnetic fields are making us sick. Power lines, cell phones, wireless internet, radio and microwaves all cause cancer. This is fact and we all know this is true even if we never like to talk about it. My cell phone gets hot when I have it up to my head for more than 5 minutes. I know I am cooking my brain.

Understanding what is going on here means entering a world most of us never knew existed, a world of electrical frequencies. Not just the common frequencies of the electromagnetic spectrum, such as radio waves, microwaves, visible light and x-rays, but also the frequencies of complex bodies, like a neuron firing, a brain thinking, a planet wobbling in its orbit or the atoms that make up your DNA. Until recently we thought our bodies were made of bone and muscle and organs and blood, and so on. With the developments in physics we now can see that the human body, or more specifically a living body, is also a complex electromagnetic system. Some frequencies are used to communicate between different parts of the organism whereas others are used to heal ourselves and repair damaged cells.

So here is the problem, we are constantly transmitting electromagnetic signals from cell phones, computers and satellites and picking them up with receivers, but our bodies also are acting as receivers. Long term effects are unknown but initial data

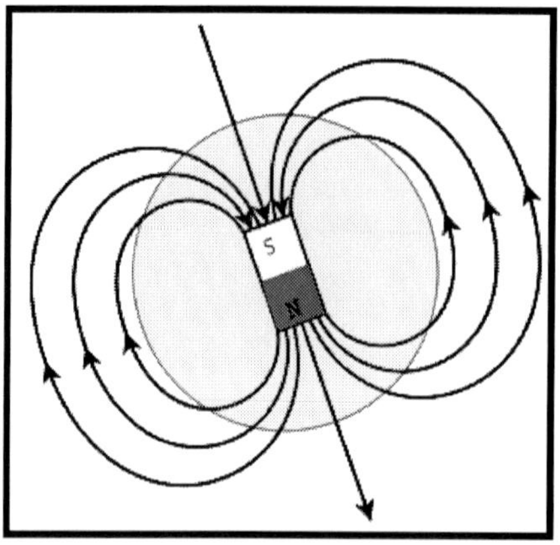

strongly suggests that these signals confuse our own cellular communication and cause interference. When the healthy signal gets confused with static from outside sources things like abnormal cell growth (cancer) can happen.

Research into the real effects of these electromagnetic frequencies (EMF) has always been hampered by interested parties who don't want the public to know, from the military, the electric plants and now the mobile phone companies. Becker's research showed that it only took 3 generations of mice exposed to EMF for the offspring to be poorly developed with stunted growth. The alarming growth in people sensitive to EMF does not make headline news and the public must be kept in the dark... until it happens to you. Like many human discoveries, the awareness of our body electric and its interactions with EMF can be used for good or bad. On the positive side, certain frequencies can be used for healing, even destroying dangerous cancer cells. However, the frequencies, and especially the mobile phone pulsed frequencies, are not beneficial. It is the difference between getting a kiss or being hit with a hammer. When used correctly, magnetic fields can help the body. Correct use can even protect your body against harmful radiation. One inexpensive and available way to do this is with a bar magnet. These have two distinct poles, a north pole and south pole. You cannot use a unipolar magnet.

North Pole: Will produce a magnetic field that has an anti inflammation effect on the cells of the body. This is good to reduce pain and in the early stages of injury recovery.

South Pole: Will produce a magnetic field to excite or stimulate human cellular tissue. This is better used once the initial healing has started. Because speeds up cellular division you would never want to use a south pole field on a pre cancerous cell because it may trigger the cancer cells to spread.

Therapeutic use of magnets for healing is contraindicated if you have a pacemaker or any other electrical device implanted in your body. Also you need medical strength magnets. These are available from speciality suppliers and generally run a few hundred dollars each. Consider the use of magnets experimental and use them at your own discretion but I continue to see positive results everyday in the clinic and in treating my own family. Magnetism is measured in gauss named after German mathematician and physicist Carl Friedrich Gauss. Here is a list of standard magnet strengths,

- 10^{-9}–10^{-8} gauss – the magnetic field of the human brain0.31–0.58 gauss – the Earth's magnetic field at its surface
- 25 gauss – the Earth's magnetic field in its core
- 50 gauss – a typical refrigerator magnet
- 100 gauss – a small iron magnet
- 2000 gauss – a small neodymium-iron-boron (NIB) magnet
- 70,000 gauss – MRI imaging machine
- 10^{12}–10^{13} gauss – the surface of a neutron star
- $4{\times}10^{13}$ gauss – the quantum electrodynamic threshold
- 10^{15} gauss – the magnetic field of some newly created magnetars
- 10^{17} gauss – the upper limit to neutron star magnetism; no known object in the universe can generate a stronger magnetic field

A typical refrigerator magnet is about 10-50 gauss. That is too weak to penetrate the skin and unlikely to be helpful for anything more than a minor bruise. Medical magnets range in strength from 450 gauss to 10,000 gauss. The higher the gauss, the better the pain relief. Clinically I like the 2" x 4" bar magnet that provides 3900 gauss each, then I will double them up (stack two magnets together) for a very strong healing effect of 7800 gauss. In some cases I will stack as many as 4 magnets together getting over 15,000 gauss, which means deep penetration.

I always enjoy hearing about how my use of magnets is quackery. Usually I get this criticism from the medical community, the same physicians who regularly recommend MRI scans to their patients for detection of disease. Somehow they have decide that the science only belongs to them. An MRI scanner is a device in which the patient lies within a large, powerful magnet where the magnetic field is used to align atoms of the human body. This causes the nuclei to produce a rotating magnetic field detectable by the scanner and this information is recorded to construct an image of the scanned area of the body. MRI's prove that magnet fields do affect the atomic composition of the human body so to discount magnetic therapy as nonsense is unscientific. Perhaps magnets do not heal, but there can be no denying that they do alter our atomic alignment. We will leave the debate for future researchers.

Recently a family member had some knee pain and called me at the office. With all my access, to hundreds of thousands of dollars of the most advance medical therapy equipment available, what do you think they asked me for? They wanted a set of magnets! So I mailed them a set and guess what, I never got them back. Every few months a will get a call from someone at their golf club or church and they really don't want to talk to me, you know what they want? A set of magnets! Oh well, at least they are taking some responsibility for their own health.

Summary

To Relieve Pain

1. DL-phenylalanine: 1000-4000 mg twice a day
2. White Willow Bark 1000-2000 mg every 4 hours
3. Biofreeze - Every 2 hours

Reduce Inflammation

1. Devils Claw: 600-1200mg day
2. Ginger: Up to 4000 mg day
3. Turmeric: Up to 3000 mg day
4. EPA: Up to 5000 mg day

To Assist Proper Healing:

1. Amino Acids: 8 (10) Essential Amino Acids
2. RNA: Up to 1500 mg day
3. Goto Kola: Up to 1000 mg day

To Reduce Stress, Anxiety, Or Viral Component:

1. St. John's Wort: Up to 3000 mg day

Self Treatment Tools:

Medical strength bar magnets: 2" x 4" (3900 gauss each) Currently I know of only on dealer in the entire country that offers these quality magnets, Health Industries, Inc. This is Dr Richard Broeringmeyer's company (a pioneer in magnet therapy). The good doctor has since passed but the company is now run by his daughter. All of my clinical magnets have come from this company. I always use two magnets stacked on top of each other for maximum benefit. Multipolar magnets are not recommended.

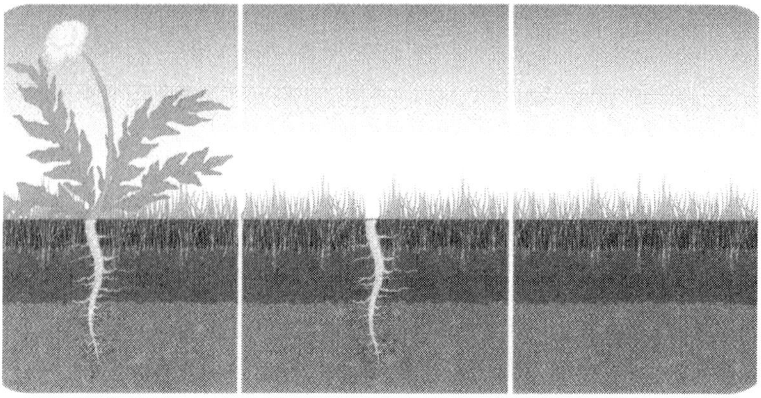

Treating symptoms only is like cutting a weed without digging up the root. The condition will usually return.

Treatments In The Clinic

The significant problems we face cannot be solved at the same level of thinking we were at when we created them.
-Albert Einstein

This chapter is a little self indulgent, please bear with me as I include descriptions of the main treatments offered in my clinic, Advanced Pain Solutions. Remember, this book was originally given to new patients as a reference and I found that most enjoyed the opportunity to learn more about how their treatments work. Many times as I was writing this book I would photocopy a few pages from the draft and hand it to the person. For the non patient reader, I hope you take the time to review this information, you may discover some excellent modalities to assist you or someone you care about towards better health.

Receptor Tonus (Nimmo Technique)

I learned this treatment while I was still in chiropractic school and it is the one I am unquestionably most experienced in. Whenever I get stuck on a tough case I always will review my original notes that I made while observing Dr. Fiscella in his St. Louis clinic. Something will always pop up to get me back on track.

Raymond Nimmo, D.C., graduated from Palmer School of Chiropractic in 1931, and set up his practice in Fort Worth, Texas. He soon became thirsty for more knowledge, so he studied other techniques. His quest brought him to the realization that what chiropractors had been taught in chiropractic colleges was not scientifically sound. He rationalized that the "bone on nerve" theory could not be substantiated by physiological facts because too many patients were being healed by manual manipulations, which did not involve bony contacts. His own chronically painful shoulder was relieved by a chiropractor who did not touch a vertebra, but corrected the problem by eliminating the hypermyotonia and trigger points (TP's) present in his body.

Being a man who questioned everything, Dr. Nimmo researched the current literature and found facts to validate his developing theory; i.e., that chronically hypertonic muscles were the cause of most of the complaints that patients presented with. He began to incorporate his research findings into his practice, and patients responded in, what seemed, a miraculous fashion.

His success attracted attention from fellow DC's who asked him to teach them what he was doing. He was a masterful teacher, beginning his lectures with the basics of anatomy and physiology. Dr. Nimmo defined chiropractic as "a branch of the healing arts that is concerned with those foci adversely affecting the function of the nervous system, which are amendable by manual methods." His constant goal in teaching was to impart what was sound neurologically and physiologically so that his theories could not be "debunked." The results he obtained were proof of the effectiveness of the "Receptor-Tonus Method" principles. Thousands of chiropractors studied his methods and changed their lives, their practices, and the health of their patients. Dr. Nimmo taught that the "bone out of place" concept, so prevalent in the chiropractic profession, actually enslaved the average chiropractor. To quote Dr. Nimmo: "Didn't they ever stop to consider that the bones are where the muscles and ligaments put them?"

He was a man 50 years ahead of his time in his thinking. He felt that chiropractors should be concerned with the functional integrity of the nervous system. In other words, if it is chiropractic to adjust a bone in the effort to restore functional integrity to the nervous system, it certainly should be chiropractic if the chiropractor directed his efforts to the factors which produce the misalignment of such a bone. To this end, a "hands-on" method, which restores the functional integrity of the body, especially the spine, by freeing the nervous system and permitting it to function normally, must be considered as a chiropractic method.

The receptor-tonus technique is a systematic approach which uses ischemic compression to remove myofascial trigger points. The doctor is instructed to search for and correct these points which bombard the nervous system and lead to subluxations by the hypermyotonia they produce in the skeletal system.

Trigger points arise from several causes, such as acute or chronic muscular overload, direct trauma, poor posture, chilling of a muscle and even emotional stress. Once a trigger point has occurred, due to metabolic stasis in the area of the TP, waste products begin to accumulate. These waste products are nerve irritants (bradykinin, serotonin, hyaluronic acid, etc.) which, in turn, produce and perpetuate pain. Due to the accumulation of waste products, the blood supply to the area is decreased and ischemia and resultant pain are felt by the patient.

The treatment consists of sustained pressure for a specified length of time, usually five to seven-seconds, but lesser time for some TP's. The pressure is applied to the patient's tolerance, always mindful of the pain threshold variances in each patient.

Dr. Nimmo's died in 1986 but his work is still instructed today by dedicated instructors like, Dr. Michael Fiscella.

This work is the basis of most trigger point therapy practiced today. Dr. Fiscella is a true master and I would encourage everyone to seek out his care when in the St. Louis area.

VAX-D Spinal Decompression

Let me start out here with a testimonial from a very special patient, Dr. Robert Channey, MD, the former assistant Surgeon General of the United States. Dr. Channey was a chronic back pain sufferer and as you can imagine, due to his position in government, he was cautious in giving any sort of endorsement. That makes his testimonial all the more powerful. Here is his story, written in his own words,

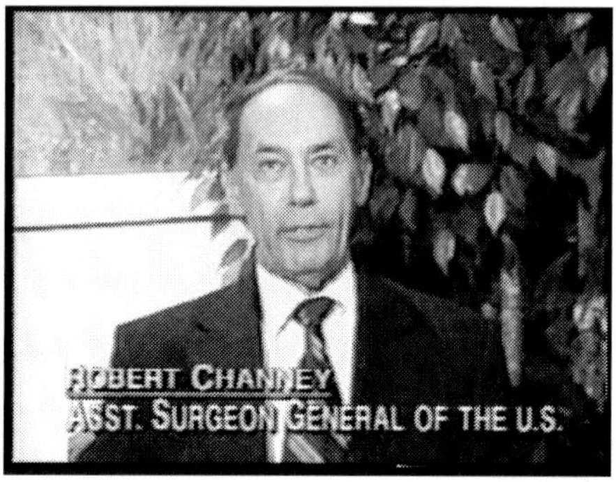

I had a back problem since 1977. We found that the discs had deteriorated at the L4-L5 and L5-S1 area. In July, I ended up with excruciating pain in my back, and this time all of the way down the left leg to my toes. It wasn't until the latter part of September that I found a program on TV about VAX-D. It looked like the thing, but I was suspicious. I called the office and made an appointment for the next day. At that time they did an extended exam on myself and recommended that I have an MRI. The MRI showed deterioration at the L4-L and L5--S1 areas. They recommended that I start on VAX-D and stay on it for 15 straight days, missing my weekends at the beach and on the boat.

I said, well it's worth a try, so I started. I was there one Saturday morning and was talking to another gentleman who was also a physician, and I said I thought this was doing well for my back but I was doubtful about the sciatic pain in my left leg. He was of the same opinion but we were going to continue on anyway. On the 27th of September, being my birthday, my family (which I have a large one) , took me for a seafood dinner down by the bay. All the way down and all the way back I could not get any relief from the aches in my back and particularly in my left leg. I continued on with treatment and after the fifteenth session I only had a slight twinge occasionally. Since that day on, I am completely free of the pain in my back and my left leg. I jog the same as I used to, as I did last evening, not a very long one, down to the park and back. I cut the lawn, I'm back without any pain at all, and I've got to say that VAX-D was the thing that did it for me.

- Dr. Robert Channey MD
Former Assistant Surgeon General of the United States Health and Human Services

This testimony is framed on the wall of my clinic and his video is posted on my website. Dr. Channey is one of thousands of people that got relief from chronic back pain with Vax-D. This is in no way a reflection on me but a credit to the creator of this technology, Dr. Allen Dyer, MD, former minister of health for Ontario, Canada.

There is a problem with the way our backs are designed. Between the bones there are little cushions called discs that serve like shock absorbers in the back. In the center is jelly (nucleus) surrounded by a retaining wall of cartilage (annular fibrosis). These discs are the number one cause of all back pain among human beings. They can get injured by torque and once they get damaged they will bulge or herniate onto your nerves causing a pain. As we get older they start to dehydrate, getting thinner and more sensitive to the pressures placed on them. When someone says they have back pain because of arthritis, in most cases what they have is degenerative disc disease, a worn out disc. To make maters even worse, these discs have no proper blood supply. There are no direct vessels bringing them blood, oxygen and nutrition. So it is very hard to get them to heal and once injured most never completely recover.

The way a healthy disc gets nutrition is from motion. This is why you must keep moving, exercise like walking is of vital importance to the health of your back and your spinal discs. Of course there is a big catch 22 here. If the disc is injured, motion hurts and damaged the disc more, so the normal process of getting blood to the disc stops and healing slows to a standstill. The spinal disc is the real Achilles heel of back pain. You can try just about anything but most treatments just do not work very good. Anti inflammatories, injections, physical therapy all may give some relief but none can repair the disc. Surgery is usually the end result of a disc injury The most common surgery involves decompressing the damaged nerve. Until recently there was no real option except live with pain or have surgery. Now we know it can also be decompressed successfully with a manual therapy called Vax-D.

Vax-D, stands for vertebral axial decompression and it is the creation of Dr. Allen Dyer, MD. This brilliant man holds several patents one that includes the technology used in the common heart defibrillator. I have met him, trained with him and he is an expert when it comes to treating back pain. Dr. Dyer set out to relieve his own back pain but discovered traditional treatments had very poor success rates.

I will find a way or I will create one. -Hannibal

He assumed that because the nature of disc damage was pressure induced he could help the condition by reducing the pressure on the damaged structures. Dr. Dyer knew about previous attempts to do this with traction therapy but recognized that traction had problems with it's design. Traction would help stretch the spine but it was unable to overcome the muscle guarding reflex. The more you stretched the tighter the muscles became. This tension causes an increase in the spinal disc pressure with leads to more damage. This was the problem with my early attempts to stretch out my back on the traction table, I hurt myself because I could never overcome the muscle guarding reflex and as a result I tore my disc more.

At the time Dyer was experimenting in his boat house, using a block and tackle set up to figure out how to pull the spine strongly enough without stimulating the muscles to respond by spasm. Spasms are a defense response to protect the spinal cord from damage. Dr. Dyer found a solution using a mathematical

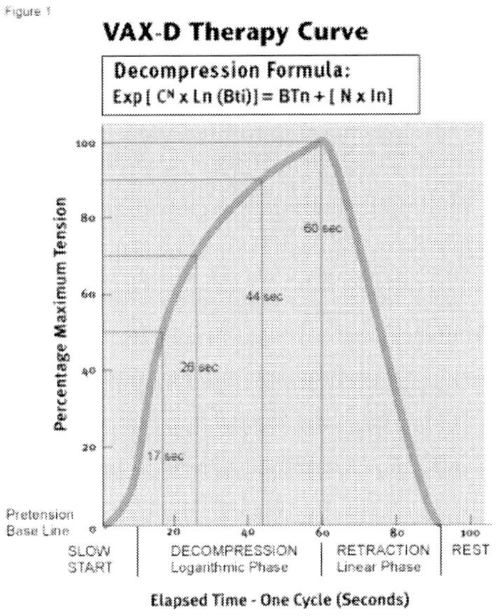

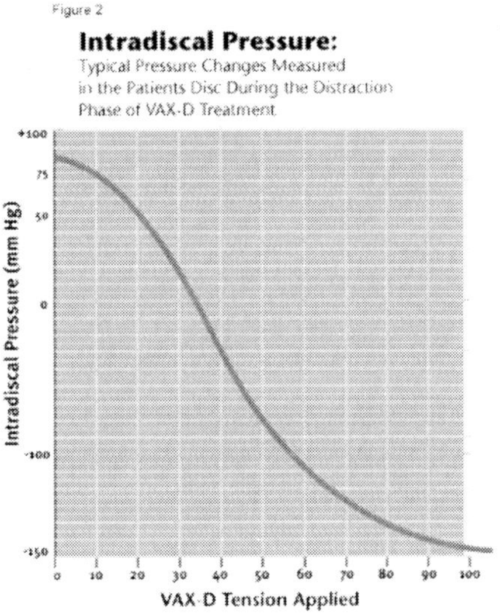

formula called a logarithmic curve. Applying pressure using logarithmic ratio tricks the brain and prevents spasm. Essentially it is a very slow, controlled pull (see figure 1.) Pistons fire using logarithmic ratios and so Dr. Dyer incorporated a piston firing mechanism in his device.

How good did it work? The pressure in a normal spinal disc is about 75 mm/Hg, when you stretch the spine with traction or by hanging on a bar you can reduce pressure down to 35 mm/Hg before it will spasm. Vax-D, with it's patented logarithmic curve treatment system can reduced pressure to negative, 135 mm/Hg (see figure 2). This means a vacuum can be created inside the damaged disc that will suck in bulges, herniations and fluid allowing it to heal naturally over a course of 20, 45 minute treatments. This has never been possible before the invention of Vax-D. The vacuum also flushed the damaged disc with blood and oxygen producing angiogenesis. This means that new blood vessels grow around the disc keeping it healthy with a fresh supply of nutrition.

70% of all true discogenic pain patients are essentially cured in less than a month. Published in Journal of Neurological Research Vol. 23, #7 Oct. 2001).

75% of patients treated with Vax-D are still pain free 5 years later. Anesthesiology News Vol. 23 #3 March 2003.

The Vax-D treatment is changing the way we treat back pain in this country. If you are suffering please accept my offer right now to come into my clinic and learn all about how this treatment that can fix your condition. You will be under some of the most experienced care in the United States. Our Vax-D associates have all been personally certified by Dr. Allen Dyer, MD and have preformed thousands of treatments. They all have passed a formal written examination and practical evaluation that includes more than 100 hours training before ever touching a patient. In addition they are all Registered Chiropractic Assistants, licensed through the State of Florida. Let's just say they really are good at what they do.

Hako Med Horizontal Therapy

The Hako Med is an electrical device that has an unusual name. If you saw how this machine looks you would think it was a robot from NASA. Standing over 3 feet tall the Hako Med has some 8 hoses coming out of it attached to suction cups. I guess it really looks more like an Octopus except for the large digital display that is constantly flashing numbers and program readouts. The Hako Med has been cleared by the FDA for a number of indications but unlike other electrical therapy devices used by physical therapists and chiropractors in the United States, this equipment has been engineered for the physician involved in clinical pain management and Neuropathy. It has a closer relationship to surgically implanted electronic simulators, but it is effectively delivered through the skin, without needles.

The Hako Med delivers electronic frequencies that can block the pain signal and heal nerves without painful injections or

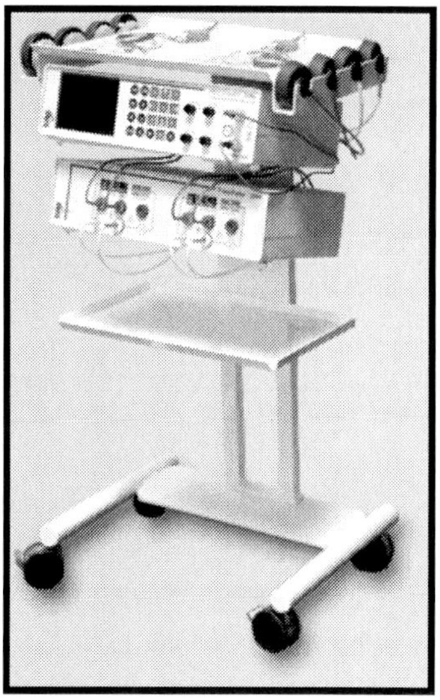

dangerous medications. Many patients will say to me it has a "feel" similar to a TENS unit but the device is much more complex and sophisticated. A TENS unit produces between 1 and 100 Hz of frequency and is able to distract the patient from their pain by vibrating the injured tissue. A Hako Med can generate frequency up to 20,000 Hz. A nerve fires at about 1000 Hz so when you expose them to these higher frequencies you can produce different biochemical effects. One way it can reduce pain is by expending cyclic adenosine monophosphate (cAMP). In other words, it uses up the chemicals that cause pain.

Dr. Hans Jurgen is the inventor of the Hako Med Horizontal Therapy device and he coined the term "multifacilitory stimulation" to describe these intracellular results and other benefits of electromedical treatments at frequencies greater than those that stimulate nerve firing. I have never met him personally but I have spoken with his son on several occasions. He lives in Hawaii where he continues his fathers research.

The Hako Med is my first line of defense when a patient comes into the clinic bent over and in severe pain. Usually after one 45 minute session they can walk upright and report 50% or greater improvement. This treatment works as effectively as a nerve block (injection) but you do not need to penetrate the skin or suffer the side effects of prescription medication. Repeated steroid nerve injections can cause osteoporosis and many other diseases. Besides most patients don't like needles. When I hurt my back I used the Hako Med several times a day as part of my rehabilitation. As I improved, I combined the Hako Med therapy with walking on a treadmill or riding a reclined bike while I breathed 5-10 liters of oxygen per minute. The results were outstanding. This device is the missing link in treating Chronic Pain syndromes like Fibromyalgia, Neuropathy, Reflex Sympathetic Dystonia (RSD) and many other nerve based disorders. I just cannot say enough good things about the Hako Med. A recent study showed that by using specific electrical frequencies it was possible to stimulate bone growth in osteoporotic patients. It seems the possibilities with this equipment is endless and it ties back into Dr. Becker's research that we discussed earlier.

Acupuncture

Most people do not now that acupuncture has been around for thousands of years and was first created by the Egyptians (some argue India). That's right, not the Chinese. I studied acupuncture under it's Asian name, Jing Luo Mai and I really enjoyed the experience. It exposed me to a hidden world of energy called Chi. Acupuncture should be considered a principle and not merely a technique. My teacher was an eccentric, larger than life man, Dr. John Amaro. Where do I begin? This guy challenged everything I had ever been taught. With Dr. Amaro there were no rules. He frequently would say things like,

Stare at a block dot on the wall until you go inside, then turn around and see where you have been.

What did that mean? Well try it and find out. He also said that the musical note of "C" represents the healing sound of the Universe. Dr. Amaro would routinely hold a C-tuning fork against a patient's skull (sphenoid bone) to induce healing. One day, noticing that I was having trouble digesting some of his esoteric ideas, he told me to buy an American Indian flute, that just happened to be keyed in C. I told Dr. Amaro I didn't play the flute and just never had the time to start learning. His reply, "Just blow into it and don't worry the flute will teach you." So I blindly purchased the native American Indian Love Flute from a Floridian craftsman, "Erik The Flute Maker". I suggest you also buy one of these instruments. Just wait and see what happens, like magic, the flute will teach you how to play and how to heal. I cannot explain, you just need to experience this for yourself. For me it was nothing short of transcendental. I know how that sounds, but still there you have it. Today I frequently will play the love flute for guests who come over for dinner and I never had any prior musical training. This is Erik's contact information,

eriktheflutemaker.com 954-424-6502 14701 SW 18 Court Davie, FL. 33325 Email us: info@eriktheflutemaker.com

Dr. Amaro taught a complete course on all aspects of Acupuncture but he believed the most powerful treatment locations were called Tsing Points or Jing Well Points. Here the energy moved close to the surface of the body and was therefore easier to manipulate. These are very small areas located on your fingers and toes. Dr. Amaro would frequently comment on these powerful points,

If what you are doing is not working or you never knew what to do in the first place treat the Tsing Points. One of my students was faced with a desperate situation where her son was in a coma in the hospital. She never knew what to do, she was at the end of her rope and there was nothing anyone could do. She sat at her sons feet and started to massage the Tsing Points, including a special point known as K1 which is located on the bottom of the foot. She did this for hours and her son woke up and can out of the coma.

These sort of stories were very common and hard to believe unless you knew the high level of integrity Dr. Amaro holds. Once I spoke with him that I was having trouble believing that the whole Chi energy system existed, he looked at me and said,

What's so hard to accept? Look at an ultrasound machine, it works by hitting a quartz crystal with energy that sends a message out into the 5th dimension seeking healing from a higher source. Everyone accepts ultrasound... Acupuncture? Acupuncture is easy to understand.

These sort of philosophical explanations went on all day long, I have an entire Moleskin dedicated to his brilliant ramblings. Many of his teaching are reproduced in my upcoming book on miracles. Many times it seemed that Dr. Amaro was playing with me, testing to see how strong my faith was. At times I felt like the young student in the movie The Karate Kid and Dr. Amaro was Mr. Miyagi. If you are able to take his course do it, you will learn a lot about being a healer and as a side bonus he will also teach you acupuncture.

So, in between Dr. Amaro showing me photographs he personally took of Qi Gong masters levitating and newspaper articles featuring him treating a baby white tiger with acupuncture, I did learned a great deal. He taught me about the human energy field. How when we are born the energy runs a certain way, up the Conception Vessel but when we die it reverses. He told me it is a waste of time to fear death because we have already done it. He said don't worry, your energy will remember what your ego has forgotten. Again, I always thought this was cool stuff even if it was a little beyond my comfort zone. I think that was his idea. One day Dr. Amaro walked into the class room and started showing slides of artist Alex Grey's work.. This are large colorful pictures of naked people with massive amounts of swirling energy fields dancing around them. Although some of it maybe a little uncomfortable for most people I believe it is the best material representation of what energy medicine is all about. A great place to start understanding this other world is to buy Alex Grey's mind blowing book,

Sacred Mirrors The Visionary Art Of Alex Grey

There is nothing I can say here to match the experience of these images, they will alter your reality. I visited Grey's store/temple/shrine/ yoga studio, while I was in New York visiting my friend Dr. Michael Gillispie. We walked around the paintings and I had a spiritual experience that forever changed how I see other humans. This change did not just happen in my mind, I physically, optically, see people differently. This enlightenment has helped my clinical abilities and opened doors where I never knew there were even openings. Suddenly the world seems like a much more interesting place to visit. Now I am inside that "black dot" Dr. Amaro spoke about and I am looking out at where I have been.

So after years of study and certification you may want to ask me, how does Acupuncture work? I cannot tell you, I can only show you. But perhaps you will find comfort in of the following two attempts. First, a little known fact about an acupuncture needle is that it creates an electrical charge when pushed into the human body. The needles are stainless steel with the handle made out of a second, different metal. In the presence of an electrolyte solution, (human tissue) the two metals generate a charge. Research has shown that even very small charges can increase the production of endorphins in the human brain. These chemicals relieve pain and as I mentioned earlier are more powerful than morphine. There are several good medical studies done on acupuncture that prove it is a useful tool for back pain and even digestive problems and they basically use this explanation. Of course it is completely incorrect. This reminds me of the title of Bob Frissell's completely insane but interesting book,

Nothing In This Book Is True But It Is Exactly The Way Things Are.

So in that same spirit I offer a completely untrue explanation that is exactly how acupuncture really works.

When we place needles into the body these thin wires act as small antennae designed to attract the power of the universe into areas of the body that require attention. Sometimes energy is drain off and sometimes it is added in. The Universe decides. I always like to think of acupuncture like making a phone call (long distance) back home to have a good talk with family that I have not spoken with for a long time. The key term here is "connection" or "reconnection".

From my experience patients who receive acupuncture get better faster. So I use it daily and just accept the modality. I guess Dr. Amaro would be happy because I finally have developed faith. Something he told me I would need if I ever wanted to become a great healer and not just a technician. Realizing that we cannot know everything is part of the human experience. According to science, bees should not be able to fly because a bee must move its wings roughly 200 beats per second, which is 10 or 20 times the firing rate of it's nervous system. I guess no one ever told a bee about science. I always think about those early scientists insisting that the world was flat or more recently the statement that it was impossible for a human to run a 4 minute mile. Then in 1954 Roger Bannister ran the mile in 3:59.4 minutes and suddenly months afterwards several people did it. We must be careful not to dismiss useful gifts like acupuncture simply because we have not yet developed the technology to objectify the data. Don't undervalue things you cannot see because you are not elevated enough to understand. A bee can fly and acupuncture works. Remember,

The frog in the well knows not of the great ocean.

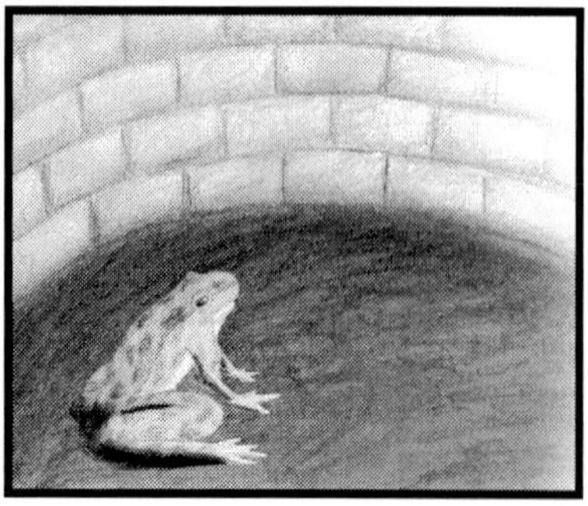

Auriculotherapy

This is a system of brain therapy that often gets confused with traditional acupuncture. It uses the external ear to identify and treat dysfunctions of the body by stimulating specific points in the ear. Auriculotherapy has recently become popular for treating addiction disorders like eating and smoking. Results come from stimulating the nerves that innervate the ear with micro-current electricity. These nerves are very unique and are known in medicine as cranial nerves. Being the most powerful nerves in the body they communicate directly with the brains higher centers and have control over just about every human function. There are 12 cranial nerves in total but 4 of them

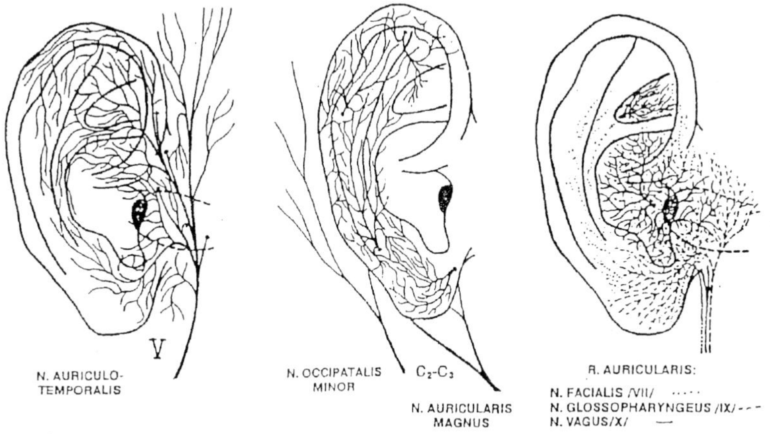

Figure 1: Nerves of the Auricle and Their Topography.
1. auricular-temporal nerve, formed by the mandibular ramus of the trigeminal nerve (V); 2. major auricular and minor occipital nerves, formed by the nerves of the cervial plexus (C2-C3); 3· auricular rami of the facial nerve (VII)- dots; glossopharyngeal nerve (IX)- dotted line and vagus (X)- continuous line.

have been identified to innervate the ear. The Glossopharyngeal nerve IX, Trigeminal nerve V, the auricular branch of the Vagus nerve X, and the Occipitalis minor nerve (cervical plexus) C2.

Let me explain how this works, for example, the stomach point on the ear correlates with the auricular branch of the vagus nerve. The vagus nerve has more branches than any other cranial nerve and some go to the stomach. The chemicals that are released in the brain as a result of this treatment are hormones, so I will cover this in more detail later when we talk about balancing the hormone system. Auriculotherapy can help anyone that is sick, regardless of the condition but I like using it specifically for addiction based disorders. In my opinion, Dr. Jay Holder of Miami Beach, Florida has done outstanding work in this field and although I am only a Neophyte I have seen lives changed with this work. I use a small device called a Stim-Plus to generate the treatment current. Because it is so simple to administer auriculotherapy it is easy to discount it as not very powerful but don't. This treatment alters the body's most powerful nerves and can help many chronic conditions.

Chiropractic

I have modified and combined many healing treatments over the years, just like when I created Budoshin Jitsu, to make them more effective. But regardless of what I study or practice, I am always first and foremost a Chiropractor. It is with pride and honor I include this brief history of my profession.

The actual profession of chiropractic, as a distinct form of health care, dates back to 1895. However, some of the earliest healers in the history of the world understood the relationship between health and the condition of the spine. Hippocrates advised,

Get knowledge of the spine, for this is the requisite for many diseases.

Herodotus, a contemporary of Hippocrates, gained fame curing diseases by correcting spinal abnormalities through therapeutic exercises. If the patient was too weak to exercise, Herodotus would manipulate the patient's spine. The philosopher Aristotle was critical of Herodotus' tonic-free approach because, he made old men young and thus prolonged their lives too greatly. But the treatment of the spine was still crude and misunderstood until Daniel David (D.D.) Palmer discovered the specific spinal adjustment. He was also the one to develop the philosophy of chiropractic which forms the foundation for the profession.

I am not the first person to replace subluxated vertebrae, but I do claim to be the first person to replace displaced vertebrae by using the spinous and transverse processes as levers...and to develop the philosophy and science of chiropractic adjustments.
-D.D. Palmer, Discoverer of Chiropractic.

D.D. Palmer was born in Ontario, Canada, in 1845, He moved to the United States when he was 20 years old. He spent the years after the Civil War teaching school, raising bees and selling sweet raspberries in the Iowa and Illinois river towns along the bluffs on either side of the Mississippi River. In 1885, D.D. became familiar with the work of Paul Caster, a magnetic healer who had some success in Ottawa. D.D. moved his family to Burlington, near Ottawa, and learned the techniques of magnetic healing, a common therapy of the time. Two years later, he moved to Davenport and opened the Palmer Cure & Infirmary.

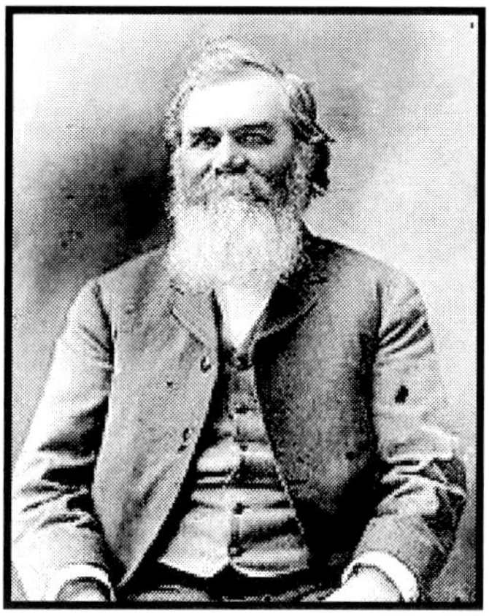

On September 18, 1895, D.D. Palmer was working late in his office when a janitor, Harvey Lillard, began working nearby. A noisy fire engine passed by outside the window and Palmer was surprised to see that Lillard didn't react at all. He approached the man and tried to strike up a conversation. He soon realized Lillard was deaf. Patiently, Palmer managed to communicate with the man, and learned that he had normal hearing for most of his life. However, he had been over in a cramped, stooping position, and felt something pop in his back. When he stood up, he realized he couldn't hear. Palmer deduced that the two events that the popping in his back and the deafness had to be connected.

He ran his hand carefully down Lillard's spine and felt one of the vertebra was not in its normal position. "I reasoned that if that vertebra was replaced, the man's hearing should be restored," he wrote in his notes afterwards. With this object in view, a half hour's talk persuaded Mr. Lillard to allow me to replace it. I racked it into position by using the spinous process as a lever, and soon the man could hear as before.

Over the succeeding months, other patients came to Palmer with every conceivable problem, including flu, sciatica, migraine headaches, stomach complaints, epilepsy and heart trouble. D.D. Palmer found each of these conditions responded well to the adjustments which he was calling "hand treatments." Later he coined the term chiropractic -- from the Greek words, Chiro, meaning (hand) and practice, meaning (practice or operation). He renamed his clinic the Palmer School & Infirmary of Chiropractic. In 1898, he accepted his first students. Although he never used drugs, under Palmer's care fevers broke, pain ended, infections healed, vision improved, stomach disorders disappeared, and of course, hearing returned.

Often surprised at the effectiveness of his adjustments, D.D. Palmer returned to his studies of anatomy and physiology to learn more about the vital connection between the spine and one's health. He realized spinal adjustments to correct vertebral misalignments, or subluxations, were eliminating the nerve interference causing the patients' complaints. At first, even though it proved to be a successful way of healing the body, chiropractic adjustments were not readily accepted. Years after Harvey Lillard's hearing was restored, the news media delighted in vilifying the pioneer chiropractor, whom they labeled a "charlatan" and a "crank on magnetism."

The medical community, afraid of his success and discouraged by its own failure to heal diseases, joined the crusade and wrote letters to the editors of local papers, openly criticizing his methods and accusing him of practicing medicine without a license. D.D. Palmer defended himself against the doctors' attacks by presenting arguments against the medical procedures of vaccination and surgery. He also cautioned against introducing medicine into the body saying it was often unnecessary and even harmful.

In 1905, the medical establishment won a minor victory when they conspired to have D.D. Palmer indicted for practicing medicine without a license. He was sentenced to 105 days in jail and was required to pay a $350 fine. Only after serving 23 days of his sentence, did he pay the fine. From 1906 to 1913, D.D. Palmer published two books, "The Science of Chiropractic" and "The Chiropractors Adjuster." He died in Los Angeles at the age of 68.

Luckily D.D. had a son, Bartlett Joshua, who was as enthusiastic about chiropractic as his father and who continued his father's work. Bartlett -- or B.J. as he is now known -- is credited with developing chiropractic into a clearly defined and unique health care system. In 1902, B.J. graduated from the Palmer school started by D.D., and before long, with his wife and fellow graduate Mabel, was helping patients and taking on more responsibility for the school and the clinic. He also was instrumental in getting chiropractic recognized as a licensed profession.

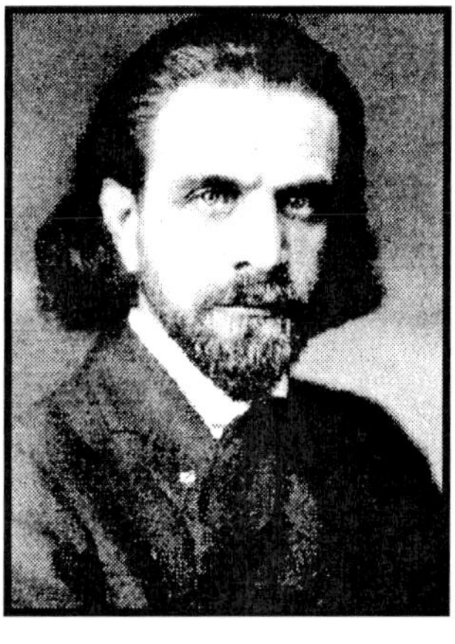

Although the profession has advanced tremendously since the days of D.D. and B.J., the basic tenets and understanding of chiropractic as a drug-free method of correcting vertebral subluxations in order to remove nerve interference still stand.

In the state of Florida, it is a written law, that only a Chiropractor is legally acknowledged to have the training and the skill to locate and correct the subluxation.

I always find it funny when a patient tells me their medical doctor said they do not need chiropractic because they do not have a subluxation. Since the state law says a medical doctor cannot diagnose a subluxation I doubt if the MD really knows what he is talking about. Anyone who studies the effects of mechanoreceptor pathways on pain relief would be doing some form of spinal manipulation on all their patients regardless of diagnosis. So why don't they? Please read on.

Medicine Vs Chiropractic

For those who may have forgotten, or for those who never knew, organized medicine spent decades and millions of dollars trying to discredit and destroy chiropractic. Today the vestiges of this suppression are still found on fringe web sites that ignore the body of peer reviewed research supporting chiropractic care. In October 1976, Chester Wilk, D.C. and four other chiropractors (one later dropped out) filed suit against the American Medical Association. The Wilk suit also named many of the nation's other most prominent medical groups such as the American Hospital Association, the American College of Surgeons, the American College of Physicians, and the Joint Commission on Accreditation of Hospitals.

The suit claimed that the defendants had participated for years in an illegal conspiracy to destroy chiropractic. On August 24, 1987, after endless wrangling in the courts, U.S. District Court judge Susan Getzendanner ruled that the AMA and its officials were guilty, as charged, of attempting to eliminate the chiropractic profession.

In 1987, following 11 years of legal action, a federal appellate court judge ruled that the AMA had engaged in a "lengthy, systematic, successful and unlawful boycott" designed to restrict cooperation between MDs and chiropractors in order to eliminate the profession of chiropractic as a competitor in the United States health care system. During the proceedings it was shown that the AMA attempted to:

- Undermine Chiropractic schools
- Undercut insurance programs for Chiropractic patients

•Conceal evidence of the effectiveness of Chiropractic
•Subvert government inquires into Chiropractic's effectiveness
•Promote activities that would control the monopoly that the AMA had on health care

This was upheld by the 7th United States Circuit Court of Appeals. The AMA offered a patient care defense; however, data from Workmen's Compensation Bureau studies served to validate chiropractic care. Specifically, studies comparing chiropractic care to care by a medical physician were presented which showed that,

Chiropractors were twice as effective as medical physicians, for comparable injuries, in returning injured workers to work at every level of injury severity.

The settlement of the suit included an injunction order in which the AMA was instructed to cease it's efforts to restrict the professional association of chiropractors and AMA members. The AMA was also ordered to notify it's 275,000 members of the court's injunction. In addition, the American Hospital Association (AHA) sent out 440,000 separate notices to inform hospitals across the United States that the AHA has no objection to allowing chiropractic care in hospitals. Since the court findings and conclusions were released, a growing number of medical doctors, hospitals, and health care organizations in the United States have begun including the services of chiropractors.

Today numerous research studies and various government inquiries have resulted in increasingly widespread recognition of chiropractic, and generally support the efficacy of chiropractic treatment. Unfortunately many people are not aware of how Chiropractic was misrepresented only a few years ago.

21st Century Chiropractic

My approach to chiropractic is a unique combination of tradition and modern technology. I use the traditional skill of palpation to locate subluxated joints that are pinching nerves. This is more of an art than a skill and must be practiced daily to be maintain. In chiropractic school we would place a human hair in telephone book and see who could find it under the most pages. Very hard, try it yourself. I also use a traditional device called a Nervoscope. This heat sensing instrument will indicate places in the spine that may be subluxated. Many times this will correlate with the palpation findings. Finally, I will always take an x-ray of the patients spine to look for rotations and areas of degeneration and disc space loss, all indications of subluxation.

Once the problem areas have been identified a specific chiropractic adjustment is preformed to correct the subluxation. In theory, one adjustment is all that is ever needed to correct a subluxation however muscular imbalance, created from years of subluxations, usually will pull the joint back out of alignment and cause the subluxation to reoccur. Many times it is therefore necessary to adjust the lesion several times, each adjustment helping the subluxation hold a little longer until it stays in place. Exercise, physical therapy, stretching, good diet and a healthy work environment can all help your subluxation hold but only a chiropractic adjustment can correct the them.

There are several ways to adjust a subluxation. For years I have used the traditional method of hands on spinal adjustment but rarely use it anymore. Over the last ten years I have discovered a better way to correct the spine that involves no popping or cracking. I use an "Arthrostim" device to place a controllable force directly into the joint I want to move. It produces a perfect adjustment every time and because it is an instrument I can record the exact pressure used to make the correction. This provided reproducible results. Patients

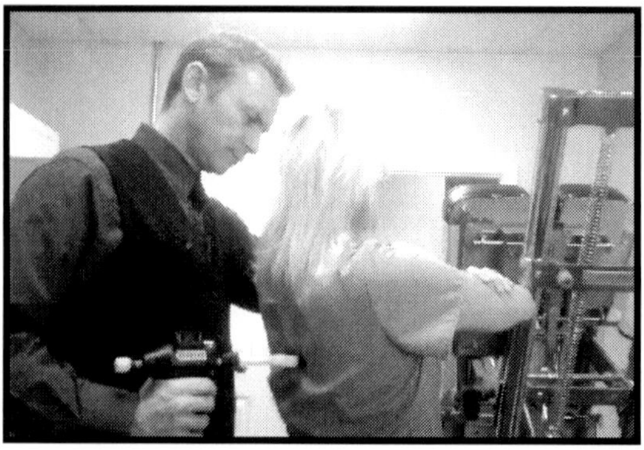

love it. I have never had a person go back to twisting and popping once they have experienced the arthrostim.

I also like to use a pelvic blocking technique developed by osteopath, Dr. Major Bertrand DeJarnette. These are wedge shaped blocks that are placed under the sacroiliac bones. Pelvic blocks use gravity to pull the joint into place without force. Just a few minutes lying on these wedges will correct most pelvic misalignments.

It only takes about 3 minutes for a skilled chiropractor to locate and adjust a subluxated spine. There is nowhere else in healthcare that a person can gain so much benefit in such a short period of time. If you are not seeing a chiropractor once a month to have your subluxations removed, do it. If you have been to a chiropractor and had a bad experience, I understand, there is good and bad in all professions. Trust me, there were guys while I was going to school I would never let touch me. I assume they are out there somewhere in practice and maybe you went to one of them. Before you give up I would encourage you to at least let me show you the difference. If you understood the benefit to your entire body that a chiropractic adjustment can provide, you would have subluxations removed from your spine before they had a chance to develop into arthritis, herniated discs or spinal stenosis. My entire family gets regular chiropractic, and not by me, we go to a local chiropractor and we pay for care, just like anyone else. It is that important for a healthy life.

Fascial Therapy

The fascia is a complex network of connective tissues that holds the muscles and organs in place. If you have ever seen an animal that has been skinned then you will recognize what fascia looks like. It's that thick, shiny, white coating over the muscles. The "grizzel" of your steak or chicken that is too tough to eat. What you may not realize is that the fascia surrounds every muscle, gives structural support to the organs and wraps around the brain and spinal cord. It is literally everywhere in the body. Being thick and strong the fascia can restrict movement patterns. If

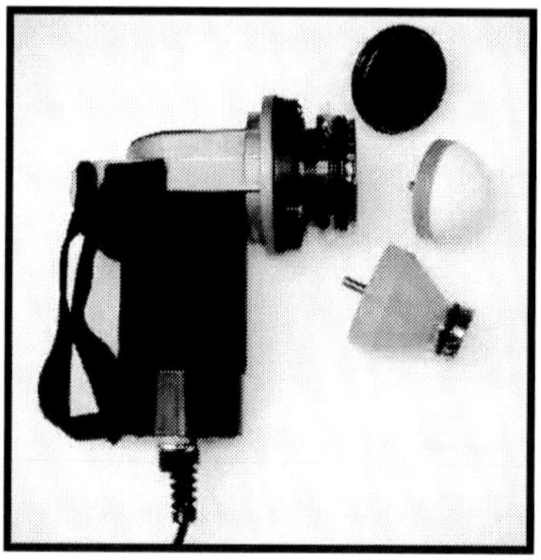

the fascia is bound up and too tight, the muscles of the body function in an imbalanced manner. Getting fascia to move correctly is hard work.

When I first started out in practice, I used a method of massage known as Rolfing to treat patients with fascial dysfunction. But Rolfing is painful to the patient and requires much effort from the doctor. So much effort that at the end of the day I sometimes wondered who was the doctor and who was the patients. Of course the Universe was listening and then one day, I was at a used bookstore in St. Petersburg, Florida and picked up Dr. Andrew Weil's book, "Spontaneous Healing." In the book Weil casually mentions an osteopath Dr. Robert Fulford as the "healing magician of our time," a doctor who could successfully "treat problems other doctors could not solve." Now that sounded interesting. What I discovered was the missing piece of my problem with treating the fascia. In the 1940's Robert Fulford DO, developed his own individual system of therapy. Fulford's many years of clinical experience convinced him that,

The fascia would never be free by hand alone.

He believed the physician needed a motorized tool to fully release restrictions. The tool that he spoke of is the modern, "Vibracussor" made in the USA by Impac Inc. The company is owned by Ed Miller, who I might add is sincerely dedicated to the Chiropractic profession. Ed really helped me get these important tools when I first started out and had no money and a student credit history. More than any other piece of equipment the Vibracussor has changed the way I practice. It allows me to get deeper into the body without activating any nociceptive, pain receptors. Patients love the Vibracussor because it feels good while making long term changes in their structure. I am almost embarrassed to admit this but it does as good a job as my hands and in some cases better. You just cannot get deep enough with your hands when treating the Iliopsoas or Iliolumbar Ligament. 30% of all the miracles I see come from using this device. If you are suffering from a condition that just won't heal make sure you devote time to treating the fascia, in most cases it will be the missing link.

Diowave 30 Watt Class 4 laser

I have said on several video interviews that if I could choose only one modality to take from my office and use for the rest of my life it would be the Diowave laser by Technological Medical Advancements. Why? Because I can use it on every condition and make at least some positive difference. These are the magic wands of health. They have been proven, 100% of the time, in multiple, clinical experiments, to increase your Mitochondria's production of Adenosine-triphosphate (ATP). More ATP means more energy and more energy means more resources available for healing.

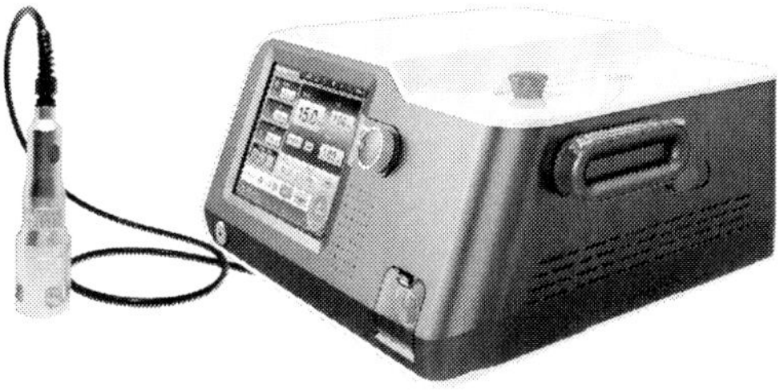

In 1967 a few years after the first working laser was invented, Endre Mester in Semmelweis University in Budapest, Hungary experimented with the effects of lasers on skin cancer. While applying lasers to the backs of shaven mice, he noticed that the shaved hair grew back more quickly on the treated group than the untreated group

All light is composed of photons. Photons are small packets of light energy—in the form of waves— with a defined wavelength and frequency. Photon energy is able to more effectively penetrate the skin and underlying structures, therefore accelerating the healing process. Light travels at a constant speed and oscillate up and down as it moves forward. However, all light is not the same. It is measured in wavelengths, with each wavelength of light representing a different color of the spectrum. The number of oscillations per second represents the frequency of each wavelength; shorter waves have a greater frequency than longer waves. Laser energy is coherent (well-ordered photons), monochromatic (single-color) light energy. When produced as a narrow, bright beam. Laser light holds its intensity until it is absorbed by a medium (the body). When applied to an organism, Laser light, tuned to specific wavelengths and frequencies, stimulates metabolic processes at the cellular level.

Studies have shown that when tissue cultures are irradiated by Lasers, enzymes within cells absorb energy from laser light. Visible (red) light and Near Infrared (NIR) are absorbed within the mitochondria and the cell membrane. This produces higher ATP levels and boosts DNA production, leading to an increase in cellular health and energy. When applied as treatment, therefore, Lasers have been shown to reduce pain and inflammation as well as stimulate nerve regeneration, muscle relaxation and immune system response.

Lasers have no effect on normal tissues, as photons of light are only absorbed and utilized by the cells that need them.

Role of Chromophores

Chromophores are components of various cells and sub-cellular organelles which absorb light. Laser stimulation of Chromophores on mitochondrial membranes incites the production of ATP resulting in:

- Increases cellular energy levels
- Allows pain relief
- Accelerates cellular healing

Clinical studies and research using laser therapy technology indicate the following beneficial effects of laser therapy on tissues and cells:

Anti-Inflammation
Laser therapy has an anti-edemic effect as it causes vasodilation, but also because it activates the lymphatic drainage system (drains swollen areas). As a result, there is a reduction in swelling caused by bruising or inflammation

Anti-Pain (Analgesic)
Laser therapy has a high beneficial effect on nerve cells which block pain transmitted by these cells to the brain and which decreases nerve sensitivity. Also, due to less inflammation, there is less edema and less pain. Another pain blocking mechanism involves the production of high levels of pain killing chemicals such as endorphins and enkephlins from the brain and adrenal gland.

Accelerated Tissue Repair and Cell Growth
Photons of light from lasers penetrate deeply into tissue and accelerate cellular reproduction and growth. The laser light increases the energy available to the cell so that the cell can take on nutrients faster and get rid of waste products. As a result of exposure to laser light, the cells of tendons, ligaments and muscles are repaired faster.

Improved Vascular Activity
Laser light will significantly increase the formation of new capillaries in damaged tissue that speeds up the healing process, closes wounds quickly and reduces scar tissue. Additional benefits include acceleration of angiogenesis, which causes temporary vasodilatation, an increase in the diameter of blood vessels.

Increased Metabolic Activity
Laser therapy creates higher outputs of specific enzymes, greater oxygen and food particle loads for blood cells.

Trigger Points and Acupuncture Points
Laser therapy stimulates muscle trigger points and acupuncture points on a non-invasive basis providing musculoskeletal pain relief.

Reduced Fibrous Tissue Formation
Laser therapy reduces the formation of scar tissue following tissue damage from cuts, scratches, bums or surgery.

Improved Nerve Function
Slow recovery of nerve functions in damaged tissue can result in numbness and impaired limbs. Laser light will speed up the process of nerve cell reconnection and increase the amplitude of action potentials to optimize muscle action.

Immunoregulation
Laser light has a direct effect on immunity status by stimulation of immunoglobines and lymphocytes. Laser Therapy is absorbed by chromophones (molecule enzymes) that react to laser light. The enzyme flavomono-nucleotide is activated and starts the production of ATP (adenosine-tri-phosphate), which is the major carrier of cell energy and the energy source for all chemical reactions in the cells.

Faster Wound Healing
Laser light stimulates fibroblast development (fibroblasts are the building blocks of collagen, which is predominant in wound healing) in damaged tissue. Collagen is the essential protein required to replace old tissue or to repair tissue injuries. As a result, Laser Therapy is effective on open wounds and burns.

I will frequently use laser in combination with other modalities. If you are getting a chiropractic adjustment in my office you may have 10 minutes of laser afterwards to help it hold better. If someone is seeing me for weight loss and we are reviewing their diet, I would recommend a laser session to them to increase fat loss. How about a weekend warrior suffering from a herniated disc? He sees me for Vax-D spinal decompression but while he is on the table I would radiate his low back with my laser.

An effective way to use a cold laser is systemically. Instead of treating a specific part of the body, like a sprained ankle you can also use it over major blood arteries. I use the carotids at the sides of the neck, the aorta above the bell button, the iliac arteries on the insides of your leg and the popliteal arteries behind each knee. I will radiate the arteries for 10 to 20 minutes depending on how sick the person is and what I am trying to achieve. Now don't get me wrong you can still treat the ankle, I just find a systemic approach produces better results.

Of course there are many lasers on the market and they all produce light so what is the difference? Well in my opinion it is all about strength. While all lasers will produce light energy most are not powerful enough to penetrate deeply into the body structures that need to be treated. The Diowave will get up to 8 inches depth, which means I can access tissues like the spinal discs. 99% of lasers on the market will not get energy past the surface layer of skin. Also the Diowave laser is 30 watts. That means it produces 3 joules of energy per second of use. Since you need 20,000-30,000 joules (laser energy) to really make a change in damaged tissues I can treat a patient in about 15 minutes. Other, less powerful lasers (most are under 10 watts) would require up to an hour to produce the same results. I guarantee

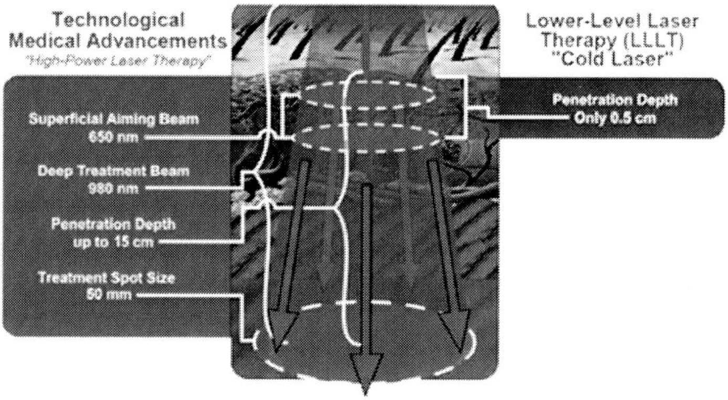

DIOWAVE DEEP PENETRATING LASER THERAPY is the key to achieving results that is more far - reaching and faster than all cold lasers..

you that no doctor is going to spend an hour treating you with laser... so the patient will never get enough joules to make a lasting change in thee clinics. Educate yourself on these concepts if considering laser therapy.

Perhaps the most dramatic example of how effective a laser can be for healing comes from personal experience. In my profession I am talking all the time. Usually during a single week I may give 15-20 hour long consultations. One day after a busy week I noticed my voice seemed squeaky. In the days that followed it started getting worse. Months later, it had not gone away and I would lose my voice after speaking for only 5 minutes. I saw an ENT specialist and he looked at my throat by putting a camera up my nose and dropping it down. Interesting experience. He said I had vocal cord nodules. These are like callouses on your voice box that form when the sides of your throat keeping slamming together. In the specialist own words, "They are painful, they bleed and they won't ever heal as long as you keep talking". His solution was to remove them with surgery. As an ironic twist they use a thermal laser to burn off the nodules.

I was not very excited about throat surgery but I had read about how nodules can turn cancerous and I was worried. This is a good example of practicing what you preach. I told the specialist I would try to heal the nodules naturally and avoid the surgery. He smiled and said sure, whatever. I know he didn't believe me. I could tell he thought I was a jerk because I was rejecting his expertise and challenging his prognosis. In retrospect, I shouldn't have done this but sometimes ego does get the better of us. So I decided to take my own medicine and the big gun for this job was going to be my Diowave laser. The vocal nodules healed completely in 4 weeks. I am not joking when I say that I could have a successful clinic doing nothing but treating vocal cord nodules. I do not know of any better way that is so non invasive. If you are a professional singer seek out the Diowave laser and save your career.

Now sometimes when I talk too much and I feel my throat getting sore I will administer a good 10 minute session of laser and it prevents any problems with my throat. This is a good example of using laser technology in different ways. Laser is here to stay, now if I could just get my flying car.

DDS 500 Orthotic Brace

More than 90% of chronic back and neck pain is caused by damage to the spinal discs. The spinal disc is a cushion that acts as a shock absorber between your spinal bones. When placed under torque the disc can squish out of shape, tear and put pressure directly on the spinal nerves. The largest spinal nerve is the Sciatica nerve, that runs into your buttocks and down your leg.

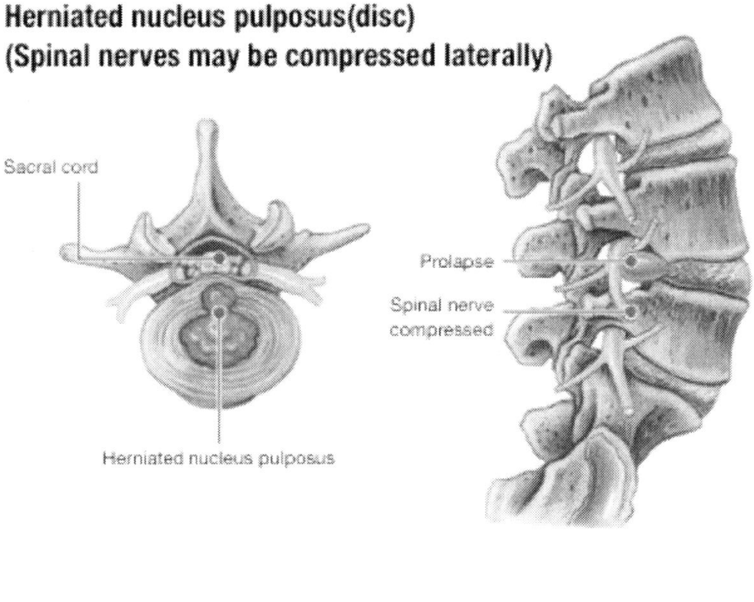

Over time if this pressure is not released it can damage the muscles and cause weakness, numbness, tingling and eventual problems walking and/ or using your bladder or sexual organs. Spinal nerve damage is a serious problem and one that needs to be treated before permanent damage occurs.

New Technology

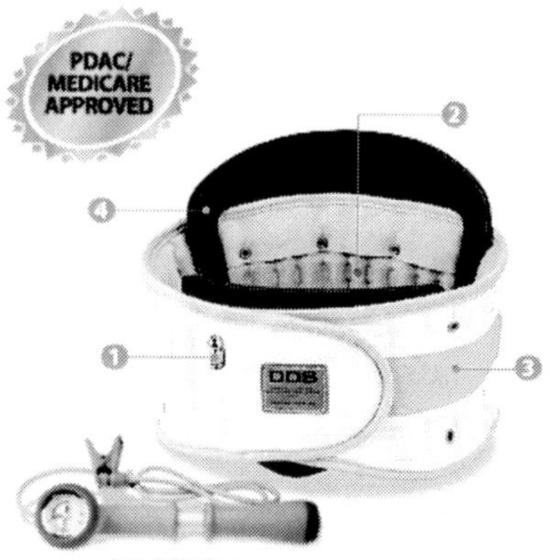

Recently advances in spinal orthotics has shown much promise in solving spinal disc injury. The new Disc Disease Solutions Brace (DDS) provides the standard support of a traditional back brace but has the added benefit of decompressing the spinal discs. The process is simple, DDS acts to provide traction between the lower part of the ribcage and the upper part of the hip creating weight-bearing forces away from the lower back. By increasing the intervertebral disc space, pressure applied on the nerve root is relieved, thereby eliminating pain while assisting active rehabilitation. The vertically expandable columns create a virtual support beam providing spinal decompression fro the lumbar vertebrae. Disc Disease Solutions will speed up your recovery and help you enjoy daily activities that were once too difficult.

The DDS is thin, lightweight and can be worn discretely under clothing allowing you to preform daily activities such as driving, walking and standing for long periods of time. Active people can enjoy sports and other leisure activities pain free. The device is PDAC approved and covered under most insurance plans including Medicare for little to no out of pocket expense. Currently there are over 2 million physicians and patients using this technology to treat back pain and sciatica.

Treatable Conditions

Herniated Disc, Bulging Disc, Sciatica, Lumbar Acute/ Chronic Sprain, Spondylosis, Lumbar Facet Syndrome, Spinal Stenosis, Degenerative Disc Disease, Post Operative Lumbar Fusion, Compression Fracture in the Lumbar Region, Failed Surgery-

Syndrome, Spondylolisthesis, Low Back Pain of Physical Origin or Obesity, Congenital Weakness in Waist.

In our clinic we provide many different types of braces but the DDS is our most popular. We are a Medicare DME provider and I am a state licensed Orthotic Fitter CF(o) so you are guaranteed of getting the right type of brace and the correct fi

Summary

Advanced Clinical Treatments

1. Receptor Tonus (Nimmo)
2. Vax-D (Vertebral Axial Decompression)
3. Hako Med Horizontal Therapy
4. Acupuncture
5. Auriculotherapy
6. Chiropractic Spinal Adjustment
7. Fascia Therapy
8. Diowave laser
9. DDS 500 Decompression Brace

and don't forget your love flute from Erik!

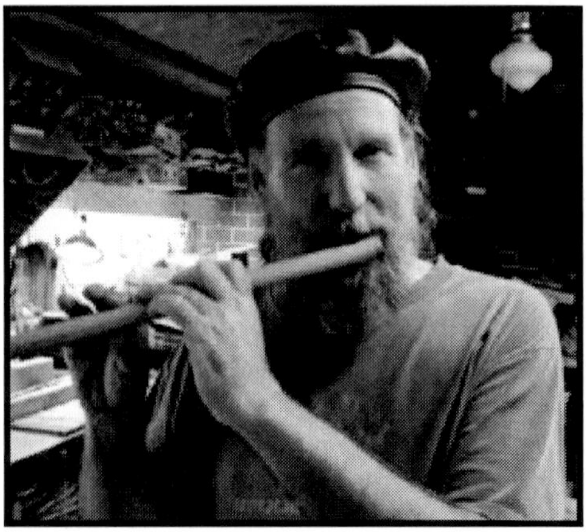

eriktheflutemaker.com
954-424-6502 14701 SW 18 Court Davie, FL. 33325
Email us: info@eriktheflutemaker.com

Step Two: Promote Detoxification

Healing is a matter of time, but it is sometimes also a matter of opportunity. - Hippocrates

The Liver

Your liver is a big filter that cleans your entire body and it is the most important organ for detoxification. Imagine never cleaning a furnace or a water filter, you must keep your body's detoxification system running perfectly or you will get sick. In addition to cleaning the blood your liver is also involved in building new tissues (anabolic activity) and breaking down old ones (catabolic activity). The liver also stores glycogen which is used for energy. Traditional Chinese Medicine (TCM) views the liver as the "General" of all the organs which works to mobilize the forces of blood to support "qi", the life force itself.

Many diseases that you would not consider associated with the liver have been found to involve faulty detoxification. Autism, for example, shows abnormal liver profiles with high levels of toxins present in the children's blood.

Patients with arthritis have high amounts of toxins in their blood that are not getting removed by the liver. One such toxin is called Guanidine and it is caused by constipation and cellular damage. Guanidine is very alkaline so when it gets into the blood stream it forces calcium out of the body fluid to restore pH balance. As a result of this extra calcium being available we see arthritic calcifications like bone spurs. This is so common that I had stopped running liver profile tests on my arthritic patients because it is 100% positive all of the time, instead I just start them immediately on a detoxification program and give them liver support supplementation.

Two important acids, linoleic acid and linolenic acid are of no benefit to us unless our liver can convert them to arachidonic acid. A person with a degenerative disease like, muscular dystrophy, multiple sclerosis or spinal stenosis has a bad liver and cannot make this conversion. This means they are deficient in polyunsaturated fatty acids. These fats are used to build protective tissue around your nerves like insulation on electrical wires.

Anyone with degenerative disease should also be very careful to avoid using products containing aluminum because it destroys this phospholipid material that protects the cell. So when you use an aluminum based deodorant it penetrates the skin into the nerve cell where it destroys its protective fat sheath and causes a neurological short circuit that stops the person from perspiring. The body continues to grow fat around the nerve and aluminum is constantly applied to destroy that protective covering. Does this make sense to you? Please avoid aluminum products. Once it gets into your system it is hard to remove and usually must treated with chelation. Taking 1500-2000 mg of Glucosamine Sulfate helps maintain nerve insulation health, but most people think it is just for joint pain.

In history there is an old say that all roads lead to Rome but in functional medicine all roads lead to the liver. Many times when I am over whelmed by a patient's condition because they are just so sick and I am unsure where I should start, I will always begin at the liver. I have a picture of the liver with it's biochemical pathways hanging in my study as a constant reminder how important it is. I know that by helping the liver and promoting detoxification I can help any condition.

Fasting

Give your body a break from food will allow it to self clean. I personally to fast one day every week, I go from Saturday night after dinner and do not eat again until Sunday night. I will drink water during my fast and although this is not recommended I sometimes will use a little green tea, because of the caffeine, to help get me through longer fasts (7-10 days). A weekly fast can keep you healthy but if you are sick longer fasts are required to detoxify the system. There are many very good books on fasting and my personal favorite is,

Fasting and Eating for Health: A Medical Doctors Program For Conquering Disease by Joel Fuhrman.

Dr. Fuhrman is the real deal, he practices what he preaches. While I don't agree with everything he recommends, I do acknowledge him as an authority on fasting. His book gives much evidence to suggest fasting is healthy and dispels many myths associated with fasting such as the risk of hypoglycemia. Fortunately the science behind fasting is very simple. Your body's main source of fuel is glucose (sugar). When you first stop eating your body looks for sources of glucose to maintain itself. The liver stores about 100 grams of glucose (glycogen) and so the body will start using these reserves as fuel. This will only last about a day and then it will run out. So the body starts to break down your fat tissue to get fuel. The problem is that there is just not enough energy available from this along and so it also starts to break down muscle tissue to get the energy it needs. You need to break down about a pound of muscle tissue a day to meet your body's requirements for glucose.

This is not such an attractive proposal. Naturally if this continued you would not last very long, as your body literally eats itself to death. Here is the good news, on about the third day (second in women) of fasting the liver begins to generate a large supply of ketones. As ketone levels rise in the blood they complete with glucose as the primary fuel source. Eventually they win and the brain, heart and muscle tissues all start using ketones as fuel instead of glucose. Now muscle wasting slows down to a minuscule rate and we get a maximum breakdown of fatty tissue, toxins and unnecessary growths. This is known as ketosis and you can easily determine when this happens by using a ketone strip, bought at the local pharmacy.

Once in ketosis you will not waste away anymore, instead all your extra material, like fat, tumors and dead cells will be burned off as fuel. The ultimate detoxification. The ultimate weight loss program. Although fasting is a great tool I recommend if you only fast while under the care of a trained physician. There can be several complications. First you must be sure that you are healthy enough to handle the stress of a fast. I will always do a complete physical including EKG and stress test before allowing a patient to fast. Furthermore, in some people they are not able to switch over to using ketones. This means that they continue to burn glucose as fuel even after fasting for two or three days. This is dangerous because they continue to breakdown muscle (a pound a day) for energy. This individual is not fasting by starving. Under these conditions the internal organs will be permanently damaged and eventually the person will expire. Very dangerous. The best way to avoid this is by using ketone test strips and if you do not go into ketosis by the third day end your fast. I have had people literally break down in tears, when after the third day, they had to end their fast because they failed to get into ketosis.

I went to Dr. Stokes because I have had back pain for most of my life. I was overweight, pre-diabetic, high blood pressure and tired all the time. As Dr. Stokes started to relieve my back pain he mentioned he had developed a program where it was possible to lose a pound or two a day and clean the system of toxic waste. After some tests I started my fast. I cannot tell you how excited I was to see the purple ketone strips on the second day. I felt inspired. I fasted for 15 days and lost 25 pounds. After the fast Dr. Stokes introduced me to a specialized diet that would maintain my weight and keep me healthy. Amazing. My blood sugar levels are now under 100, I have perfect blood pressure and tons of energy. I would recommend that anyone really interested in changing their lives speak with Dr. Stokes.

-Ken P, Cape Coral, FL

What To Start Doing Right Now

The following supplements have been tested to improve just about any chronic condition by making the liver healthier.

1. Trimethylglycine (TMG): Take 3000 mg daily

There are many disorders and diseases that are related to the liver. Hepatitis, Fatty Liver and Cirrhosis all come to mind. Like I already mentioned the liver is important in every body function. One challenge a doctor faces when trying to heal the liver is that many patients are already on so many prescription drugs that it is almost impossible to give them something that will not react with the prescriptions and cause side effects. This is why I love TMG to rebuild the liver. If you are suffering from any liver based illness this is absolutely required. TMG is primarily found in beets, so it is perfectly harmless regardless of your condition. Studies for this product are amazing. It can prevent cirrhosis, it can physically help regenerate a damaged liver and it can reduce homocysteine in the system. Take 3000 mg everyday for 6 months and then re test your liver. If needed do a full year at this dosage. Once you have healed take 1000 mg a day as a maintenance dosage for liver health. I take TMG every day and so does my whole family. This is the one essential super supplement.

2. Glutathione: Take 400-1000 mg daily

Glutathione is the most important component of the liver's detoxification system. There are not many products that I would say can make a miracle but this is one. Glutathione preserves

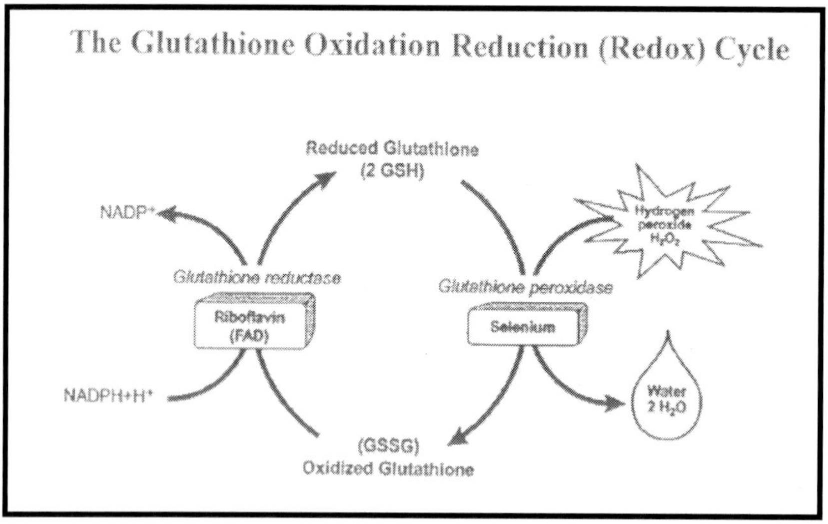

brain tissue from damage. It has the power to halt the onset of Parkinson's disease and should be "the" first line therapy for all degenerative diseases. If you just don't know where to start, start with glutathione and you cannot go wrong. I use glutathione on a regular basis and so do all my patients. It is a natural product so it cannot be patented by the big drug companies so you will hear very little about it but do your own research.

Made very simple, glutathione takes dangerous chemicals in your body and makes them harmless by way of the glutathione oxidation reduction cycle. I remember when I first saw the before and after video footage of Parkinson's patients who had received glutathione I was in a state of shock. These patients went from hardly moving to prancing up and down the hallways, waving to the camera and hardly shaking. If you watch these videos you will investigate glutathione and make it a part of your health care program.

This is a miracle supplement but oral administration of Glutathione does not get into the blood stream, it breaks down in the digestion process. There are currently only two ways to get Glutathione into your system, via intravenous therapy or with a nebulizer. Intravenous is ideal but not for self treatment. Most patients can learn to use a nebulizer and therefore it is the pre-

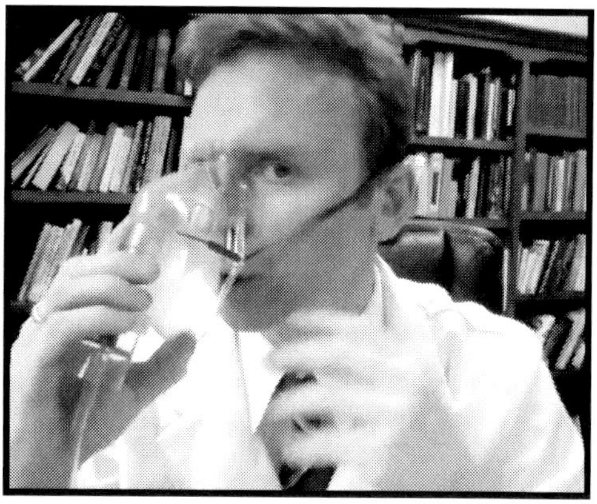

ferred method. Recent studies suggest that although some potency is lost with nebulization therapeutic dosages of Glutathione will still reach the blood stream. The best glutathione for nebulization is buffered with sodium bicarbonate.

The sodium bicarbonate renders the resulting solution roughly the same pH as the lung. If not buffered, GSH in solution will have a pH of about 2; with the buffer, the solution will have a pH of about 6. So this is the very best product available. With this particular product, which provides 200 mg of GSH per capsule, an isotonic solution is formed with approximately 3 cc's of water per capsule. Some patients can tolerate hypertonic solutions and are able to use less water per capsule. The water should either be sterile, or boiled or distilled water which has been cooled to approximately room temperature. This is done to prevent the growth of waterborne bacteria such as Pseudomonas Aeruginosa within the solution. It is really best to mix a solution when ready to nebulize and it is no longer usable after 5 hours post mixing. When inhaled, the solution will produce an odor which is inoffensive to most but offensive to some, for it has a sulfurous smell. The goal is a 400 mg treatment mixed with 6 cc's of sterile water solution twice a day for acute care.

You will need a prescription to get a nebulizer, contact my clinic if you have trouble getting these materials. Glutathione is a natural product that has incredible properties for detoxification but you cannot take nebulizer Glutathione if you suffer from any breathing disorder like asthma or you are allergic to sulphur. Always see a physician before trying nebulized Glutathione. I have seen this product completely change a person in less than 30 days. Absolute miracles. It takes work but Glutathione is turning heads, even in the medical community. The Mayo Clinic is using this method of administering Glutathione for the management of COPD with incredible results.

Glutathione Facts

• It is found in almost all living cells. The liver, spleen, kidneys, pancreas, and the lens and cornea, have the highest concentrations in the body.

• It is a powerful antioxidant and thus neutralizes free radicals and prevents their formation.

• Has an important role in immune function via white blood cell production and is one of the most potent anti-viral agents known.

• It is one of the strongest anticancer agents manufactured by the body.

• It is used by the liver to detoxify toxins including formaldehyde, acetaminophen, benzpyrene and many other compounds.

• It is an antioxidant necessary for the protection of proteins; is involved in nucleic acid synthesis and plays a role in DNA repair.

• Glutathione levels decrease with age. It is involved in cellular differentiation and slows the aging process.

• Protects the integrity of red blood cells.

• Glutathione is involved in maintaining normal brain function.

Therapeutically, Glutathione is used for:

• Detoxification/Chelation
Heavy metal toxicity including mercury, lead, arsenic and cad-

mium. Common toxins that glutathione may help protect against are car exhaust, cigarette smoke, aspirin and alcohol. Pesticide and industrial chemical exposure. Steroids. Bacterial toxins (Clostridia difficile). Pharmaceuticals (very long list that need to be detoxified by the liver)

• Immune enhancement: 1-3 g per day. This is especially effective against clostridium in the GI. It helps prevent translocation.

• Psoriasis

• Diabetes mellitus: Especially in ketosis as DM patients will generally excrete increased amounts of sulfur containing amino acids.

• Liver disease including cirrhosis and fatty liver disease caused by alcohol.

• Ulcers intestinal or stomach

• Aspirin or phenacetin overdose (useful for rheumatoid arthritis patients or chronic pain sufferers on 8 or more aspirin/day)

• Hematological conditions: myelofibrosis, acute leukemia, chronic myelocytic leukemia, lymphoma, polycythemia vera

• Alcoholism

• Before radiation therapy to strengthen the system.

• Cataracts

• Parkinson's disease, Alzheimer's Disease, ALS (Lou Gherig's disease), Multiple Sclerosis, other neurologic conditions including Autism/Pervasive Developmental Delay and Chronic Kidney Failure.

The Coffee Enema

There is another way you can increase your body's own production of Glutathione and that is a coffee enema. All the body's blood passes through the liver every three minutes. So the ideal retention time of a coffee enema is 15 minutes, that way we can detoxify the blood system 5 times per session. When exposed to caffeine the hemorrhoidal blood vessels dilate and in turn dilates the livers portal veins. So we get this big increase in flow which in turn stimulates the production of Glutathione. This is an enzymatic catalyst that attaches itself to toxins in your body and makes them available to be removed as waste. In studies done with mice liver detoxification increased by 600% and the small bowel detoxified by 700%. These are big numbers. I learned about the value of coffee enemas by studying the works of Dr. Max Gerson, MD. I would highly recommend anyone interested in learning more about this healing modality read,

The Gerson Therapy: The Proven Nutritional Program For Cancer and Other Illnesses by Charlotte Gerson and Morton Walker, D.P.M

Charlotte Gerson runs a treatment center across the border where they are reversing terminal cancer with nutrition and detoxification protocols. When I first read about Gerson Therapy I was skeptical and then one day a patient came into my Fort Myers office seeking relief from back pain. Again, it seems that the Universe was listening. During my comprehensive clinical history the patient mentioned they been diagnosed with terminal cancer 10 years ago. His doctor told him go home and get his life in order which is doctor talk for prepare to die. He went to the Gerson clinic and continued the protocols for a year. Today he is 100% cancer free. He has great story and told me that as he was doing the Gerson Therapy, he started feeling so good that he had to keep reminding his wife that he was supposed to be dying. She kept making all these plans for the future and he was told he would not be around. Then patient told me that at one point he remembers distinctively stated to his wife, "You know honey I just don't think I feel much like dying anymore." and of course he never did. It is a great story that I am happy he shared with me. So part of that protocol was the coffee enema which I am presenting here in simplified format,

Coffee Enema Instructions
You can get enema bags at any drug store, they look like a hot water bottle with a tube coming out of the end.

First prepare the coffee:
1 quart distilled water in a pot
6 heaping teaspoons of ground organic coffee.

Let the mixture boil for 3 minutes and simmer for an additional 15 minutes. Cool to body temperature and strain through a coarse cloth or fine strainer. Do not prepare the enema coffee as though you were brewing coffee. The coffee bean is very high in potassium, which is absorbed into the colon and is an "anti-cramping" agent. Normal brewing does not release the potassium, so the resulting coffee is deficient in this all-important mineral.

Now administer the enema. There are two types of enemas, the retention enema and the cleansing enema. The cleansing enema should be done first. This is a regular enema with distilled water and no coffee to void the colon of all waste. One you have emptied your colon then, add distilled water to the coffee solution and place in the enema bag. Insert the lubricated tip into the rectum, while lying on your left side. After the fluid is in, clip the enema tube and remove it. Retain the fluid for 15 minutes. Roll to the center, lift pelvis up to get the coffee to the transverse colon and roll to the right. The primary action of

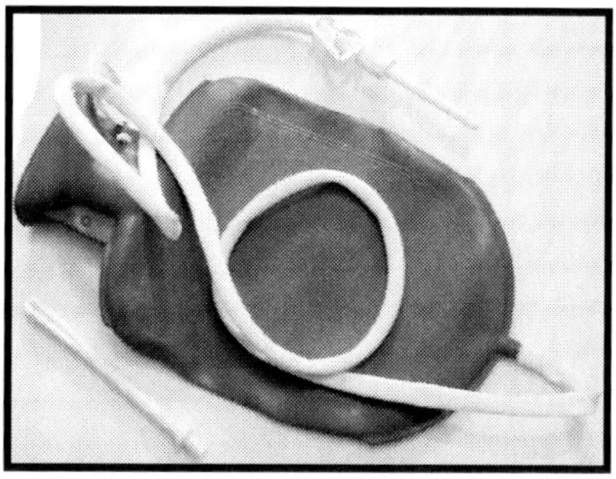

the retention enema, which is held in the body for about 15 minutes, is to help rid the liver on impurities. The caffeine goes through the hemorrhoid veins directly into the portal veins and into the liver.

The body should be lying down on the right side, with both legs drawn close to the abdomen and breathe deeply. Massage your colon. After 15 minutes, sit on the toilet, stand up, move around and try to expel again. At first you may only be able to hold the coffee for 3-4 minutes. Build up your retention times over daily enemas.

If someone is very sick I will tell them to do these daily until I start seeing changes, eventually I tell patients to do one of these every few week or at least one a month depending on their intake of bad food, alcohol etc. A coffee enema can be used whenever you want to clean out your entire system. It is a powerful tool that everyone can use.

Alcohol

When alcohol is consumed, it passes from the stomach and intestines into the blood, a process referred to as absorption. Alcohol is then metabolized by enzymes, which are body chemicals that break down other chemicals. In the liver, an enzyme called alcohol dehydrogenase (ADH) mediates the conversion of alcohol to acetaldehyde Alcohol is damaging to the liver and every system of the body. There is not anything useful or positive about this poison. It has the same effect on blood vessels as smoking, most people do not realize that alcohol will first open up the blood vessels but later produce a rebound effect causing severe vasoconstriction. Blood is your life line and you need to keep it flowing. You cannot be serious about living to your maximum potential if you drink alcohol. I know there is a big psychological attraction to social drinking but it is not good for you. If the liver is busy detoxifying the alcohol it will have little energy left over for making you healthy. So again to just reinforce my professional opinion, there is no safe or beneficial amount of alcohol for a person to consume.

My aunt Joanie was a slim beautiful woman who slowly degenerated over the course of 15 years and eventually die in her 50's due to alcoholism. On her death bed she would not see anyone except my mother. In her last hours she confessed how wrong she had been and how she had painfully wasted her life because of alcohol. If you or someone you love is an alcoholic get them help before it is to late. There is nothing healthy or beneficial about alcohol regardless of what manufactures try to convince us.

Smoking

If you smoke for whatever reason you need to quit right now. Smoking is the single most damaging habit anyone can do to their health. I can easily tell if a person smokes by looking at his complexion. The smoker will have a gray skin tone that comes from an accumulation of toxins. Because blood vessels are constricted when you smoke waste cannot wash out of your cells and instead it just builds up and eventually changes the color of your skin. No blood flow means no oxygen and that means no energy or nutrition for healthy function. So if you smoke you will die sooner than you should, it's that simple. The guy who smoked his whole life and lived to be 100 years old would have lived to be 120 years old, get the point? Smoking not only destroys your own health but has the potential to destroy the health of those around you, so it is socially irresponsible. In my clinic, many times, I will refuse to accept a patient until they have committed themselves to stop smoking. The chemicals found in cigarettes also have a detrimental effect on your cellular health. Along with lung cancer, which is fairly obvious, these chemicals damaged essential DNA that will lead to an eventual breakdown of just about every bodily system. That's bad, right? Anyone who has watched someone they love died of emphysema will testify that it is a painful and horrible death. Essentially patients drown as their own blood fills their lungs and breathing becomes impossible. We know that smoking constricts arteries and reduces blood flow in the body. This reduction in blood flow slows down the natural healing process of the damaged tissue. It is a major obstacle in promoting the bodies natural healing ability. A less known but equally important side effect of smoking is the effect on the brain. The addictive properties of tobacco alter brain chemistry reinforcing neurological pathways that can lead to chronic pain. More on this later but for now just be aware that smoking has a profoundly negative affect on every aspect of your health.

I have never witnessed a patient die from giving up smoking. You do not need patches, gums or prescribed medications. You just need to grow up and take responsibility. I speak from first-hand experience. I smoked throughout my 20s as I was studying to be a doctor. Believe me, I see the irony. In truth smoking is just a choice you make. I quit cold turkey, it was not easy but it was possible. I did it and you can too. There is no excuse to smoke. I can administer some auriculotherapy treatments to your ear that will release certain chemicals in your brain designed to make you feel less withdrawal from quitting but you will still have to make the decision. Once you stop smoking you can heal the damage to your body with specialized therapies. In about a year your body will start functioning again, your lungs will heal and you will look and feel 10-15 years younger. Glutathione, administered through a nebulizer, is very effective in helping clean the lungs. Right now, today, at this very moment throw away your smokes and never light up again. It is that simple.

Oxidata Test

One test I like to run on all patients coming into my program is the Oxidata Free Radical Activity Test. This is a urine test that shows levels of free radical activity in the body. It works by measuring the distant end of the polyunsaturated fat chain were aldehydes form as result of free radical attacks. We use urine because aldehyde activity is more concentrated there. Let me put it another way for you,

The Oxidata Test is 50 times more sensitive than blood serum free radical testing.

Free radicals are formed with almost every biochemical reaction in the body. They are a byproduct that the body has to get rid of. This test can show how effectively the body is quenching these free radicals. If there is a high levels present this could be an indication that the bodies detoxification system is malfunctioning. This is another very easy test and many patients enjoy performing this at home and testing family members. Turmeric was mentioned earlier as something to combat inflammation but it is also a home run when it comes to controlling oxidation.

Summary

To Clean The Body Of Toxins:

1. Fast: Daily up to several weeks
2. Trimethylglycine (TMG): Take 3000 mg daily
3. Glutathione: via nebulizer up to 1000 mg day

Self Treatment Tools:

1. Coffee Enema: Up to twice a day
2. Avoid Alcohol
3. Stop Smoking

Testing:

1. Oxidata Test

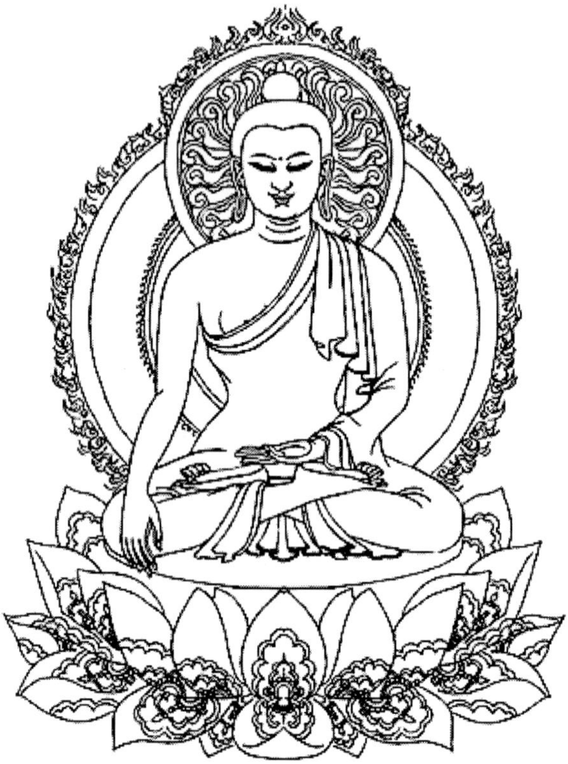

One of his students asked Buddha, "Are you the messiah?"
"No", answered Buddha.
"Then are you a healer?"
"No", Buddha replied.
"Then are you a teacher?" the student persisted.
"No, I am not a teacher."
"Then what are you?" asked the student, exasperated.
"I am awake", Buddha replied.

Step Three: Strengthen Digestion

A man has often more trouble to digest food than to get it.
-Proverb

The human digestive system is a complex series of organs and glands that processes food. In order to use the food we eat, our body has to break it down into smaller molecules that can processed and then excreted as waste. The digestive system is essentially a long, twisting tube that runs from the mouth to the anus, plus a few other organs like the liver and pancreas that produce or store digestive chemicals. I picture the food slowly moving throughout my inner body massaging and healing as it travels my core. If you don't have a similar image of food than perhaps you should reconsider what you are eating?

The digestive process begins in the mouth. Food is partly broken down by chewing and the chemical action of salivary enzymes. These enzymes are produced by the salivary glands and break down starches into smaller molecules. After being chewed and swallowed, the food enters the esophagus. The esophagus is a long tube that runs from the mouth to the stomach. It uses rhythmic, wave-like muscle movements, called peristalsis, to force food from the throat into the stomach. This muscle movement gives us the ability to eat or drink even when we're upside-down. This is why astronauts can swallow in space.

The stomach is a large, sack-like organ that churns the food and bathes it in a very strong acid. Food in the stomach that is partly digested and mixed with stomach acid is called chyme. After being in the stomach, food enters the duodenum, the first part of the small intestine. It then enters the jejunum and then the ileum which is the final part of the small intestine. In the small intestine, bile (produced in the liver and stored in the gall bladder), pancreatic enzymes, and other digestive enzymes produced by the inner wall of the small intestine help in the breakdown of food. After passing through the small intestine, food passes into the large intestine. Here some of the water and electrolytes are removed from the food. There are many different types of bacteria that lives in the large intestine. Some are useful and some are harmful. As we will learn later maintaining this balance is important for your health. The food enters the first part of the large intestine which is called is called the cecum. The appendix is connected here. The food then travels upward in the ascending colon across the abdomen in the transverse colon and then goes back down on the other side of the body through the descending colon The final part of the colon is called the sigmoid and it is here waste is transferred to the rectum where it is stored until it can be excreted via the anus.

The process of digestion is complex and we need to remember that when we eat something it will move through all these different steps exposing our bodies to either healing or harm.

Leaky Gut

Leaky gut syndrome also called increased intestinal permeability, is the result of damage to the intestinal lining, making it less able to protect the internal environment as well as to filter needed nutrients and other biological substances. As a consequence, some bacteria and their toxins, incompletely digested proteins and fats, and waste not normally absorbed may "leak" out of the intestines into the blood stream. This triggers an autoimmune reaction, which can lead to gastrointestinal problems such as abdominal bloating, excessive gas and cramps, fatigue, food sensitivities, joint pain, skin rashes, and autoimmunity. The cause of this syndrome may be chronic inflammation, food sensitivity, damage from taking large amounts of nonsteroidal anti-inflammatory drugs (NSAIDS), cytotoxic drugs and radiation or certain antibiotics, excessive alcohol consumption, or compromised immunity. A significant percentage of children with autism have increased intestinal permeability. Allergies and many other medical conditions are now being linked to leaky gut syndrome. It is always the first place I address when it comes to digestive problems. If you have a leaky gut avoiding alcohol, NSAIDS and follow the recommendations at the end of this chapter.

The Intestinal Permeability Test

As part of my 10 point examination I usually will order a blood test called Intestinal Permeability. The Intestinal Permeability Test, also called the Lactulose and Mannitol Test, measures the ability of two sugar molecules, mannitol and lactulose, to permeate the intestinal lining. Ordinarily mannitol is easily absorbed but lactulose is not. The test can help to identify malabsorption which can cause nutritional deficiency.

Increased permeability and weakness of the intestinal lining barrier, which can cause toxins and larger molecules to enter the bloodstream and lymph circulation. Once in the bloodstream, the immune system attacks these unwanted substances and it also increases the load on the body's detox system. The following has been linked to poor digestion,

- Acne rosacea
- GERD
- Indigestion
- Candidiasis

•Crohn's disease
•Eczema
•Food allergies
•Low back pain
•Sinusitis
•Rheumatoid arthritis
•Unexplained weight gain
•Abdominal Pain
•Heart Burn
•Bloating
•Anxiety
•Gluten Intolerance
•Malnutrition
•Muscle Cramps
•Pain
•Poor Exercise Tolerance
•Allergies
•Celiac Disease
•Multiple Sclerosis
•Fibromyalgia
•Autism

Gut Flora

The human body, consisting of about 10 trillion cells and carries about ten times as many microorganisms in the intestines. The metabolic activities performed by these bacteria resemble those of an organ. Bacteria make up most of the flora in the colon and up to 60% of the dry mass of feces. Somewhere between 300 and 1000 different species live in the gut, with most estimates at about 500. However, it is probable that 99% of the bacteria come from about 30 or 40 species. Fungi and protozoa also make up a part of the gut flora, but little is known about their activities.

Research suggests that the relationship between gut flora and humans is not merely commensal (a non-harmful coexistence), but rather a mutualistic relationship. Though people can survive without gut flora, the microorganisms perform a host of useful functions, such as fermenting unused energy substrates, training the immune system, preventing growth of harmful, pathogenic bacteria, regulating the development of the gut, producing vitamins for the host (such as biotin and vitamin K), and producing hormones to direct the host to store fats. However, in certain conditions, some species are thought to be capable of causing disease by producing infection or increasing cancer risk for the host.

It is of vital importance to maintain the proper balance of good and bad flora in order to promote health. People may take the drugs to cure bacterial illnesses or may unintentionally consume significant amounts of antibiotics by eating the meat of animals to which they were fed. Antibiotics can cause antibiotic-associated diarrhea (AAD) by irritating the bowel directly, changing the levels of gut flora, or allowing pathogenic bacteria to grow. Another harmful effect of antibiotics is the increase in numbers of antibiotic-resistant bacteria found after their use, which, when they invade the host, cause illnesses that are difficult to treat with antibiotics.

Changing the numbers and species of gut flora can reduce the body's ability to ferment carbohydrates and metabolize bile acids and may cause diarrhea. Carbohydrates that are not broken down may absorb too much water and cause runny stools, or lack of SCFAs produced by gut flora could cause the diarrhea.

A reduction in levels of native bacterial species also disrupts their ability to inhibit the growth of harmful species such as C. difficile and Salmonella kedougou, and these species can get out of hand ultimately leading to serious pathology such as cancer. Establishing healthy flora is the second most important step in promoting systemic health.

What To Start Doing Right Now

Dramatic improvement in health, regardless of your diagnosis, can be seen just by improving the digestion process. Here are the simplest things that will begin to heal your gut. Monitor how you feel as you take these important steps. Do not try to change your digestion over night, this will take time and you have to go slowly. Start with small dosages and work up to where you need to be.

1. Enzymes: Plant based, 1-3 capsules with every meal

An enzyme is a protein catalyst that makes possible the chemical reactions that digest our food and break it down to usable, absorbable nutrients. Enzymes are only found in living things. There are two categories of enzymes, the ones we make inside our bodies, called metabolic enzymes and the ones we get from outside sources, like the foods we eat. Cooked and processed foods are perhaps the single most detrimental deterrent of health because enzymes are destroyed at temperatures of 118°F and above. This means that almost any kind of food preparation method will destroy enzymes. Anytime you cook, microwave, fried, baked, grilled or otherwise process your foods, you subject yourself to dangerous consequences of eating enzyme deficient foods. When that happens our bodies are force to draw upon our metabolic digestive enzymes. The problem is that there is a limited supply of these backup enzymes available and depleting the supply places stress on the body. If your body is spending energy digesting your food, less energy will be available to do other things such as heart disease, burn stored body fat or delay the aging process. Eventually as your body's stores of digestive enzymes are completed, you become unable to digest certain for withdrawal. If you were to use up your supply of lactase enzymes (from eating enzyme deficient milk products) you would soon become lactose intolerant. Use up your supply of amylase (from eating too many simple carbohydrates) and diabetes could be in your future.

The goal is to ingest enzymes at every meal. There are two ways to accomplish this. You can eat a balance diet that includes raw fruits and vegetables at eat meal or you can take a plant based enzyme supplement every time you eat. Many people resolve conditions like heart burn and acid reflux disease practically overnight once they stop using up their metabolic enzyme storage. I have seen patients drop blood sugar values in less than

1 week just by adding enzymes with every meal. This is truly one of those remarkable little secrets of being healthy that everyone can do. Whenever I am out I will carry enzymes in my pocket so if I am forced to eat a meal that does not have living foods in it, I can take a few enzymes capsules. I would encourage you to do the same.

Protease, lipase, amylase and cellulase are the main enzymes to look for in a multi enzyme supplement. They represent about 80% of the market. These are made from aspergillus and grown in a laboratory setting on plants such as soy and barley. They are called plant based, microbial and fungal. Of all the choices, plant based enzymes are the most active or potent. This means they contain the highest active units and can break down more fat, protein and carbohydrates in the broadest pH range than any other source. In the United States almost all enzymes are made from a single company and then sold to various vitamin manufacturers.

I will frequently specialize a patients enzyme program to include more of a particular enzyme that they need, (sugar digestion or protein digestion specialization being the most popular) but you should just take a good multi enzyme supplement. That way you cover all your digestion needs. I am going to cover digestive enzymes extensively in step 5, including where I feel is the best source to get them from.

2. L-Glutamine: 2-4 grams A.M. and 2-4 grams P.M.

This is really great stuff and it can help with any type of lower GI problem. L-Glutamine serves two purposes, it maintains the gut barrier function and it helps with cell differentiation. By strengthening your gut barrier it prevents toxins and nasty stuff from entering into your blood stream and making you sick. This ability to modulate intestinal permeability improves the entire body's immune function. The digestive system is one place where cells are constantly being sloughed off and replaced. L-Glutamine's role in cellular differentiation serves as a great insurance policy against disorders like cancer because it makes sure that the new cells are healthy and free from defects. These high turn over areas are always areas that disease can prosper. When used with digestive enzymes it is the best defense against leaky gut syndrome.

3. FOS (fructooligosaccharides): 750-1500 mg day

If you can even say this word you will get extra credit but don't worry if you ask for FOS most people will know what you mean. This is a sugar that we cannot digest but the good bacteria in our colon eats for food. It is know as a prebiotic for that reason. The good bacteria is called a probiotic. You can naturally increase your probiotics by taking this supplement and just making sure the good bacteria that you already have are well fed. Eventually they will out number the bad bacteria. Many patients will experience gas or bloating whenever they begin manipulating their probiotic count but this is usually only temporary until your body adjusts.

4. Probiotics: Acidophilus 6 billion units per day

Lactobacteria such as acidophilus and bifidus are known as friendly bacteria and inhabit the intestinal tract, especially the colon. They are extremely important for proper digestion and excretion and responsible for maintaining proper pH balance in the colon. They also suppress the growth of bad bacteria and keep infectious yeasts such as Candida under control. Lactobacteria are destroyed by chlorinated water, antibiotics and diets high in animal protein, which support the bad bacteria. The good and bad bacteria are constantly fighting in your gut for dominance. Most people have a ratio of 20% lactobacteria to 80% bad bacteria. The correct ratio for optimum health is 80% lacto to 20% bad.

People who eat yogurt think they're getting plenty of lactobacteria into their systems, but it's not true unless they make your home everyday and consumed within 24 hours. After 24 hours the bacteria even the best yogurts began to decline rapidly leaving lactic acid which is a waste product of like the bacteria metabolism. Also if you are eating yogurt that is mixed with sugar (or fruit) the live bacteria will be compromised. The easiest and richest source of supplemental lactobacteria is cabbage. Cabbage feeds and promotes the growth of whatever friendly like the bacteria are already present in the digestive tract. It also suppresses growth of bad bacteria controls gas and reduces bowel odor. If you are suffering from stomach ulcers or want to increase good bacteria growth here is my super secret formula,

Drink 1/2 cup of freshly fermented cabbage juice times a day. In the morning blend one three-quarter cup distilled water with 3 cups coarsely chopped loosely packed fresh cabbage in a blender. Start at low speed than switch to high speed for about 30 seconds. Pour combine mixture into a jar cover loosely and let stand at room temperature for exactly 3 days. Then strain off the liquid. Immediately measure out a quarter cup and start your next batch by blending 3 cups coarsely chopped cabbage with 1 1/2 cups of distilled water and then pouring it back into the jar along with the quarter cup from the first batch. Shake and let stand covered at room temperature for 24 hours this and all subsequent batches requires a quarter cup, plus water and take only one day. Store the rest of this drink in the refrigerator and take half a cup three times per day preferably with meals discard any left over juice after 24 hours. Continue making and taking the juice daily for one to three months. The cabbage juice should be sour, slightly carbonated with and mineral taste.

Another food that will promote good bacterial growth is Jerusalem artichokes. They contain a carbohydrate called inulin which is neither digested or absorbed by humans and therefore reaches the lower bowels intact. Your good bacteria loves this stuff and it helps them multiple and grow up to be happy bugs. Heavy fiber foods such as selenium husks, carrots and sprouts also help support good bacteria by sweeping the colon clean of their competition. It is hard to consider bacteria to be good for us but the truth is we are sharing the earth and this body with millions of other creatures.

Acidophilus is the number one probiotic supplement you can buy, there are others, but start with this. Until recently I only recommended refrigerated Acidophilus because it seemed that off the shelf products were too weak. That has changed and now there are several ways to maintain the potency of probiotics without refrigeration. You need to do some research for yourself to find the product that best works for you. Always supplement after taking antibiotics to restore your natural flora. For any bowel related disorder Acidophilus is a must.

When a friend was having trouble with bad breath for years despite perfect dental hygiene he asked me what I thought. After doing a history I found out that he had undergone an extensive treatment of antibiotic therapy. Around the same time his breath started smelling. He also sufferer from constipation. I suggested a 3 month trial of enzymes, L-Glutamine, FOS, and Acidophilus. This did the job. He started producing a daily bowel movement almost right away and guess what? After about a month no more bad breath.

Obermayer Test

In the clinic I administer a simple test called an Obermayer or Indican Test. This is done with a urine sample and is super easy to preform. How easy? Many times patients will buy the test from me and go home to test their spouse or children. It shows us the presence of something called dysbiosis or unbalanced colon flora. The great thing is you can retest yourself frequently and see if your treatments are effective. Here is how it works. Tryptophan is an essential amino acid common in dietary protein that is converted to indole by the intestinal bacteria. Indole is converted to indican in the liver and is processed and excreted in the urine. The production of indican reflects bacteria activity within the intestines. Elevated levels indicate overgrowth of bad bacteria. The test uses Chloroform, HCl acid and a ferric Chloride mix ... nasty stuff so you have to be careful, don't drink it or inhale it's fumes and you will be okay. If you are interested in the Obermayer Test call the clinic for information. We typically send out several of these every week all over the country. Establishing proper digestion is the best thing you can do for allergies. Many patients have reversal of allergies almost as a secondary benefit taking these supplements.

Summary

To Assist Digestion:

1. Plant based digestive enzymes with each meal
2. L-Glutamine: 2-4 grams AM and 2-4 grams PM
3. FOS (fructooligosaccharides): 750-1500 mg day
4. Acidophilus: 6 billion units per day

Testing:

1. Mannitol Test - Leaky Gut Syndrome
2. Obermayer Test - Dysbiosis

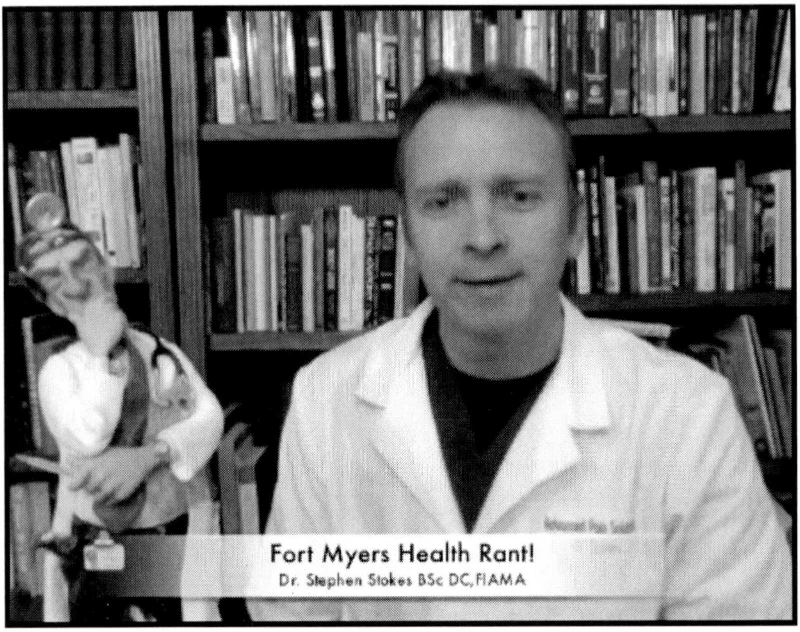

A screen shot taken from Dr. Stokes weekly your tube show, "Fort Myers Health Rant". This is a completely free educational program that promotes the 7 steps to innate healing while answering specific questions viewers may have.

Step Four: Balance Immune System

But however secure and well-regulated civilized life may become, bacteria, Protozoa, viruses, infected fleas, lice, ticks, mosquitoes, and bedbugs will always lurk in the shadows ready to pounce when neglect, poverty, famine, or war lets down the defenses.
-Hans Zinsser Rats, Lice and History (1934)

The Most Important System

The body does not have an immune system as much as it is an immune system. Systems such as the skeletal, respiratory, reproductive, endocrine and central nervous system are complete functioning systems with a clear set of organs and immune responses. For example, the stomach releases HCL to destroy ingested parasites, the spleen releases antibodies, intestinal flora destroy pathogenic microbes and the thymus releases lymphocytes. Therefore what is referred to as the immune system cannot be enhanced without enhancing the overall health of the whole body.

This is a common theme of this book and every step is designed to be completely integrated. Our immune system has 3 powerful actions at it's disposal when we are attacked by invaders. First is the initial response and I always refer to this as the army. Inflammation is a good example of this initial response. Our body sends out white blood cells to gobble up the invader and they are disposed of in the form of pus. If that is unsuccessful your immune system will create an abscess that will keep the enemy away from doing harm until it can be drained. The second response is called adaptation. Think of this as the special forces. Here your body develops a specialized group of cells called antibodies that are trained to attack specific invaders. This takes longer a little longer that the initial response but once it starts working it is very powerful. Finally, we have a third tool called the lymphatics. This is the body's massive filtering system made up of lymph fluid and nodes. It carries away dead invaders and assists the other immune players. Your tonsils are an example of lymph nodes. They swell when you are fighting an invader because the nodes are filtering the carnage of your immune system in action. This is all very complex and I am in no way giving you a course on the immune system, I just want you to understand that your body has a way to deal with things that are trying to make you sick and as long as your immune system is functioning correctly you will be healthy. Just think for a moment, how many times has someone you've known gotten sick with a cold and despite being around them you don't get it? For me, I see sick patients everyday but I rarely get sick because my immune system is healthy.

I cannot overemphasize that infectious disease is the number one threat to your health. I am seeing data to suggest that almost every known disease has a germ origin. Diabetes, fibromyalgia, back pain and migraine headaches can all be linked to the presence of infectious agents. With this in mind is it really that great of a jump to suggest that a person can catch something like back pain? This deserves further consideration. Next we will have a look at some important areas that directly relate to your immune systems health, hygiene, allergies and stomach acid.

External Hygiene

Most people realize the connection between cleanliness and disease. Today germs are more of a threat than ever before and if you don't your immune system healthy they will win. Let's start with the basics. Do you shower every day using soap and shampoo? Do you use deodorant, and keep your toenails and fingernails short and clean? Do you brush your teeth at least twice a day and keep your tongue clean as needed? Do you wash your hands before every meal and after being in public places and touching things such as doors tables and computers? How about after you use the washroom? These simple tasks make a major difference. Don't be fooled by people who say not to worry about germs. I once heard a mother tell me she purposely exposes her child to unsanitary conditions to strengthen the immune system. This is completely ridiculous.

Historically the odds of surviving a surgery more than doubled once doctors began using soap and water, just washing their hands saved many lives. So do these simple things. I always keep a bottle of hand sanitizer handy and suggest you do the same. These are just simple basics, the minimum for staying healthy. There are several things you need to have on hand always to maintain any reasonable level of health and perhaps the most important item you can buy is bleach. Make sure you wash your toothbrush and anything else you want to keep clean and a small amount of diluted bleach frequently. Put it in a spray bottle and use it on countertops that may be contaminated with germs. I will soak coffee mugs and dishes that have been used in my office in a sink full of diluted bleach once a week. In addition, I have staff wipe down all the tables, doorknobs, bathrooms and countertops everyday. If a patient known to have an infectious disease like Hepatitis, Herpes or HIV comes into my office, we disinfect immediately after they leave. The truth is we know very little about many bacteria and viruses, diseases like cancer may even have a viral component (in my opinion most diseases have a microscopic invader preventing healing), so in a clinic like mine we are always thinking about hygiene. I ask all patients right on the intake form if they have any infectious condition and then we process then accordingly.

Make sure you wash your clothes in hot water with a good brand named detergent, especially underwear and intimates. Do not use towels more than a few times before cleaning them. A wet towel can invite nasties to take up dwelling. Disinfect your shower, bathroom and toilet area since germs tend to multiple there in excess (bleach works great here as well). Trust me, if you could see what I have seen under a microscope you would clean your home everyday. Change air filters regularly, if you have them, and consider buying a portable air cleaning system especially if you live in an apartment with shared air or have animals living with you. That guy in the apartment upstairs who is always sick ... you are breathing in his germs. Stuff spreads fast.

It's a fact that most people are just not very good at cleaning themselves. Make sure you wipe your bottom with a good quality toilet paper after each bowel movement. It is even better to follow up after you wipe with the paper with a quality, "Fresh Wipe" unless you can afford a bidet which will allow you to wash the area with soap and water. If you are over weight it is really important that you devise a system to keep your genitals and rectum clean after every elimination. Seriously consider installing a bidet and begin fasting to lose weight. If you don't know about the bidet get educated. I believe it is an essential tool for anyone severely over weight. Look into it and trust me. You have keep this area clean to be healthy.

If you are prone to excess hair in the genital area keep it trimmed short and comfortable. Pubic hair, under arm hair, chest and back hair are an evolutionary throw back. The hair is designed to retain our scent in order to attract the opposite sex for mating. To an animal, this stimulates primal sex drive but for the modern human, it is not always desirable. I can guarantee you that my sweaty underwear after a 2 hour bike ride does nothing for my sex life. Extra hair will harvest germs, especially if you live in a hot climate or sweat often. Wear a clean new under shirt everyday and chose good deodorant. Do not use an antiperspirant because they contain toxic aluminum that will lead to many different sorts of neurological diseases. By the way, all antiperspirants contain some sort of aluminum, it's how they work. The rock crystals that are supposed to act as natural antiperspirants are just aluminum in various hidden forms. Avoid them. Besides you want to mask the odor and not stop the body from sweating all together. Unfortunately many natural brands found at health food stores do a bad job of masking the scent. The only brand my wife and I have found is Old Spice. They make a few different scents and some are tropical and women can get away with wearing them and not smelling like a sailor. I personally like the Old Spice original formula.

Next question, how are your teeth? I always look in a patients mouth and at their tongue whenever I have the opportunity to examine them. No, I am not a dentist but I am interested in how clean the mouth is. We know 100% the correlation between cardiovascular disease and poor dental health. Where do you think all those germs in your mouth end up? Destroying your heart valves and arteries, that's where. Brush your teeth. I carry a tooth brush in my pocket that I bought at a drugstore, it folds! I brush after every time I eat acidic or sugary foods or at the very least after each meal. I use a good quality toothpaste that I got from my dentist, not natural feel good stuff that is made from flowers, but stuff that will kill germs. Remember, we need to kill the bad bacteria while keeping a healthy environment for the good bacteria to live in. There is always a trade off. As far as fluoride is concerned I have studied the data and I use toothpaste that contains fluoride. Why? It prevents cavities, no question about it. You can make your own toothpaste using sodium peroxide and baking soda if that is your thing. Finally, do not forget to floss. Yes, it takes time, yes it hurts at first, yes it is gross. Hey it's your mouth and your heart. I frequently will rinse my mouth out at the office in between patients or chew on breath mints or sugar free gum. Right, I know sugar free gum is not good for me but neither are germs, this is one of those choices you will have to make.

When a patient comes in my office for their initial consultation and it appears that they lack what I would classify as basic hygiene or they smell of body odor, waste, animals or alcohol, my nurse will put a note on their chart and I will always take 10 minutes (okay sometimes this goes on a while longer) to discuss with them the concept of personal hygiene. I usually give them this chapter from my book to read, so if you were given this as a handout to read ... surprise! We have some work to do. Now sometimes the patient will be offended or embarrassed but that is not my intention and once they see I am sincere, most will start practicing some of these recommendations.

As a doctor, I'm an educator by default. Many times patients are unaware of how they are perceived by other people and are thankful that somebody is interested enough in their well-being to take the time and discuss these matters within a safe and private setting. Odor is a great, primal indicator that something is wrong. So if you smell funky clean yourself up inside and out. I once studied Traditional Chinese Medicine with a Dr. Pham (he was from Cambodia). He could diagnose a patient from how different parts of their body smelled. It was weird and very invasive, even a little creepy but there was definitely something to it. I know that there are dogs trained to locate patients who have cancer by way of smell so maybe old Dr. Pham was not far off. For me, I am not that sensitive in my smell but I certainly know when something stinks. Well, enough said.

This brings up another sensitive item, people living with animals. Animals have no place living with us. It was when humans started domesticating animals and living among them that many diseases began to surface. Animals are filthy, this is a fact and if you suffer from chronic illness get rid of them. If you have animals and are not sick this only means your immune system is strong (so far). I can usually tell a patients who has pet animals because they smell like a combination of dander and excrement. It is not healthy. To me, the whole idea of keeping animals as pets is weird. I know people who have children walking around in dirty clothes and shoes with holes in them but still they maintain a bunch of cats and dogs. This is simply irresponsible. Animals cost a lot of money to maintain. Can you really afford pets? Maybe you can but can you afford the illness that may come along with the animal? Not me, not my patients. Can you imaging someone slowly dying of an autoimmune disease (most diseases are autoimmune) and making their immune system also have to deal with all the germs of a pet dog or cat. Insane. If you want a group of animals buy a farm and keep them outside away from you and your family otherwise get another hobby maybe get a goldfish, that would be the most risk I would take. I know this is not going to sit well with all you animal lovers out there but please understand, I do not hate animals. I am a doctor and my responsibility to educate my patients on the truth even if it is unpopular. Animal domestication is just selfish.

If I could talk to the animals, I wouldn't because they are ****** animals. -Comedian Dennis Miller

Internal Hygiene

Keeping your external environment clean and germ free is the first step, but you must also keep clean on the inside. I will be spending time on food later on but for now I want to discuss fasting, again. It requires no cost and is available to everyone. Fasting will have a profound on both your state of health and the time you will live. That's correct, I am saying you will be sick less and live a longer life if you practice this simple ritual. It is the very best way to keep your insides clean and healthy. Now wait, don't get all discouraged and assume you know about this because you most likely don't. The goal is to fast 24 hours every 7 days. How long should you maintain the practice of fasting? The rest of your life. By not eating for a 24 hour period you will allow your body the chance to eliminate wastes and most importantly rest.

The gastrointestinal system is like a machine and every time it gets used it wears out a little more. Not eating one day a week you will be adding 52 days a year to your GI health. Impressive when you consider that the cells of your body can only divide a limited number of times before death. It makes sense to slow down this process if we want to promote health, but there is more to the story. When your body is not busy processing food it has extra time and energy to focus on other things like healing damage. This is a good thing if we are sick. So pick a day that will be easy for you, I like weekends, and have your last meal on say Saturday night and do not eat again until Sunday night, it's what my wife and I do. Drink water if you are thirsty but do not feel like you must force the issue. You will most likely not feel very good the first time you do this but you will survive. Most of the time the reason you will feel bad is because of withdrawal from caffeine, sugar and dairy but we will address these in the diet section. For now, commit to fasting one day every week. This will be the first step towards controlling your life, there is no reason you cannot do this, it is all psychology and since this is just the first step I suggest you really give it an honest try. If you refuse to even do this, you will find the more advanced suggestions impossible. As a side effect of fasting your total caloric intake will also go down and you will lose about a pound a half pound a week. In the chapter on diet I will go into detail about long fasts to lose weight and help cure many incurable diseases, for now use fasting weekly to keep your systems healthy. As you will see later fasting is the single most powerful thing you will be able to do for yourself to overcome sickness.

Food Allergy

As the years roll by I am more convinced that most chronic diseases have an autoimmune component. Diabetes, fibromyalgia, digestive disorders, headaches, arthritis, back pain... I could go on. All these conditions have been greatly helped or completely reversed when I have balanced the patients immune system. Every person's body reacts to foods differently. Therefore you need to test yourself to determine which foods cause toxic reactions in your system, you could be eating a diet that contributes to your health problems. The biggest players in this puzzle are food allergies.

Some toxic reactions to foods (also called food sensitivity or allergies) are self evident. The body responds quickly with obvious symptoms like hives, a rash, difficulty breathing, and even potentially life-threatening reactions such as anaphylactic shock. Eating a green pepper may cause bloating and lethargy. Lemons may cause headaches. Still others could avoid excess pounds if they removed eggs and soy from their diet. Without proper testing, these connections may go undetected.

However, most of the body's negative reactions to food toxicity are not so obvious. Patients often suffer through years and even decades with symptoms that they believe are unavoidable. The adverse symptoms of many toxic food reactions are often misdiagnosed or covered over with a medication, creating dependency on prescriptions rather than encouraging the body to heal.

Just like you have a fingerprint you also have a blood print. The first place to look whenever I have a patient suffering from chronic illness is for food allergies. I believe that in my clinic we offer the very best test available anywhere in the world. We test the patient's blood for 156 different foods and substances to determine exactly what they should not be eating or exposing themselves to. This information alone has completely reversed hyperactivity in children, cured migraines and helped thousands of patients lose stubborn body fat, permanently.

When I test a patient using the standard skin prick allergy test, about 5% of the population will demonstrate allergic reactions. These are immediate reactions and use the IgE model or the initial response classification. When I test patients using a delayed reaction test 90-95% of the population will have a reaction. This is an insane number! Why is this happening? One big reason is sugar. We consume more of this poison than ever before. Children are sucking back sodas, fruit juices, energy drinks, and even so called vitamin waters at an alarming rate. Sugar destroys the immune system. This is why when someone is trying to repair the immune system and eliminate the allergy you must also refrain from all sugar intake or it will not work. My personal experience with allergies has been that the patient will need about 8 weeks of complete avoidance from the food to clear a normal IgG allergy and more intense reactions may require 6 months, but that depends on your genetics and how much damage has been done to your immune system. If the allergy clears, the patient can resume eating the triggering food as long as the immune system stays balanced. Use the protocol discussed in the digestion chapter to heal the system during this period.

Please listen, this is complicated stuff and if you have a deadly reaction to peanuts, do not try any of this on your own because you could die!

Is that clear enough? See a Doctor who knows about this type of treatment. If your doctor doesn't know about testing for delayed food allergy reactions, then my guess is he or she is not going to be much help. Did I mention I am taking new patients? Seriously, please be careful.

Stomach Acid

Does allowing billions of dangerous bacteria to enter your body sound like something you are interested in doing? Let me be the one to break the bad news to you, if you are taking anti acids like Rolaids and Tums or acid blockers like Pepcid AC, Tagament and Zantac, that is just what is happening. These products reduce your body's production of hydrochloric acid (HCL). Now the problem is that many digestive problems, such as heart burn, are not being caused by too much acid but to little. With not enough HCL available the foods you eat will not breakdown. Food molecules will pass into the bloodstream undigested where they are attacked by your immune system.

The autoimmune response caused by incomplete food digestion is the basis for many diseases such as Rheumatoid Arthritis, Lupus and Crohn's. When food fails to breakdown in the stomach harmful bacteria take up residence and before you know it the bad bacteria will create an ulceration in your stomach. The ulcer causes the once beneficial secretion of HCL to cause pain because the stomach wall is unprotected. Taking an anti acid will further slows down the stomach's production of HCL which allows more bad bacteria to grow and eventually leads to a full blown autoimmune reaction.

The solution is simple. Stop taking anti acids or acid blockers and reestablish normal production of HCL. Sometimes, in cases of severe bleeding ulcers, it will be necessary to heal the stomach first before increasing your HCL. The best way to do this is with chlorophyll. The molecule is almost identical to hemoglobin with the difference that chlorophyll has magnesium and hemoglobin has iron. Chlorophyll contains all the fat soluble elements that are necessary to build the mucous membranes of gastrointestinal tract and essentially repair the ulcer. Once healed you can begin some hydrochloric acid therapy as follows,

As soon as betaine hydrochloric acid is placed in solution (stomach) the betaine and the HCL separate which makes the HCL available to the stomach. This is good for people who cannot digest protein or absorb minerals. Betaine hydrochloride also contains pepsin which is another proteolytic enzyme normally found in the stomach.

I feel that the betaine hydrochloric acid supplement made by Standard Process is one of the best available.

What To Start Doing Right Now

Okay so lets talk about getting the immune system working at it's best. These products are my personal favorites, which means they work and they are very safe.

1. Beta Glucan: 100-500 mg day

This is a chain of glucose molecules found in such foods as oats, barley, mushrooms (like the Shiitake) and yeasts. It improves

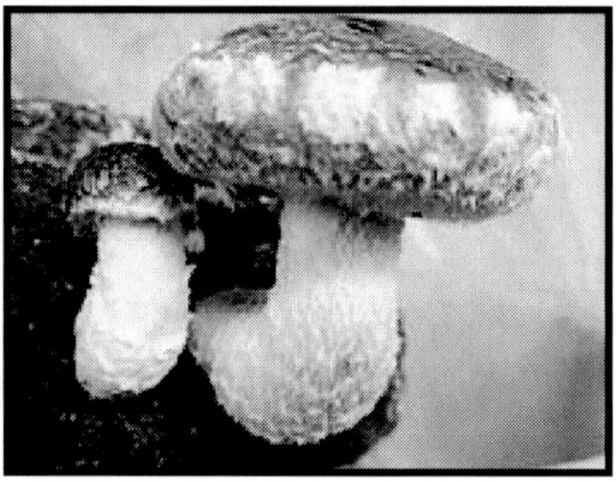

the function of your immune system and has been show to be very safe even at high dosages. For general support take 100 mg a day and for chronic diseases like cancer or diabetes take up to 500 mg a day.

Beta Glucan has also been shown to have a profound affect on insulin and blood sugar. This stuff is so powerful patients can reduce their cholesterol to the point of not needing medications. We know that statin drugs cause all sorts of bad side effects so if you suffer from high cholesterol or high blood sugar you need to start taking Beta Glucan right away. Remember that more than 80% of your immune system has it's foundation in the gut. Everything you need to do for digestion also applies to the immune system.

Chronic diseases like cancer and diabetes have viral components. The only way to help yourself is by maintaining a strong immune system and reducing exposure to all the horrible dangers found in our food and environment. People are eating out in places that are not preparing food properly and exposing them to large doses of dangerous pathogens. Our food is grown with toxic chemicals and our livestock is exposed to a multitude of disease and filth, prevention and lifestyle change is the message here. Every time you eat out there is a risk of Hepatitis. This is heavy, just think about this. That guy in the kitchen, screwing with your food, you don't know what he is doing with it or if he has a cut on his finger. My guess is that he has not read my instructions on personal hygiene, so all he has to do is not wash his hands after he goes to the bathroom and presto my friend, you are in deep trouble. If you think I am over reacting, the sad truth is I am not. Many of these diseases will not show up right away. Some are silent for years before they surface. Who really knows how this stuff is spread. Here in Florida, there was a big Federal investigation a few years ago in a small town located in the middle of the state. There were many people outside of the normal demographics contracting AIDS. Scientists started thinking that perhaps the virus had somehow mutated and was airborne. Suddenly the whole town looked like a scene from the X-Files, then just as fast as it all started everything stopped and they all went away. No one ever heard the results from the studies. All media attention just halted. To this day I don't know what happened but I think you need to be careful and don't assume everything is clean and safe, protect yourself. A strong immune system is a good first line defense, go out and buy some Beta Glucan today.

2. Echinacea: 1000-2000 mg day for up to 10 days

Most people have heard about this herb. Native Americans used Echinacea Angustifolia root and Echinacea Purpurea root to support the immune system and as a tonic. Echinacea is one of the most popular herbs in the United States. Whenever I need a very strong immune modulator I will prescribe echinacea. It works great with skin disorders such as psoriasis, acne, eczema or for any short-term treatment of infectious conditions such as influenza, colds, cystitis, and shingles, particularly those of a chronic or recurrent in nature. Quality is extremely important when dealing with echinacea because in human trials it was the alkylamides of the echinacea that was the only chemicals found in human plasma samples.

It's important to use echinacea at the first signs of infection. This is done to usually stop the infection in its tracks however if it does take hold the echinacea may not be enough. Important to remember that besides being an immune enhancer echinacea is also an immune modulator and has much value in treating many autoimmune conditions. It is not a stimulator it is a balancer and this is an important property because immune stimulators can make autoimmune diseases worse. It also has anti-inflammatory properties which make it ideal for incorporating it into many different types of condition treatments. It is definitely one of my top herbs that I use everyday. The preferred species of echinacea is angustifolia and E. purpurea. Be careful in using other types because there are may quality issues with this herb. This is one of the only supplements I do not recommend just going down to the corner store and buying because quality is so important. There are not many good companies producing echinacea. Medi-herb is the exception but as always do you own research.

Summary

Immunity Balancing:
1. Basic Hygiene Practices
2. Eliminate Food Allergies
3. Avoid Anti Acids and Acid Blockers
4. Beta Glucan: 100-500 mg day
5. Echinacea: 1000-2000 mg day for 10 days only

Delayed Food Allergy Test:
1. Immuno Lab Bloodprint

Step Five: Nutritional Deficiencies

The reasonable man adapts himself to the world; the unreasonable one persists in trying to adapt the world to himself. Therefore all progress depends on the unreasonable man.
-George Bernard Shaw

The 4 Steps To Correction

These are the most important steps in the entire program. Diet is powerful medicine and it does not require a prescription. If you do nothing else except change your diet you will dramatically change your life. Everyone is different and rarely recommend the same food to every patient, however this chapter represents the common themes. There are 4 important parts,

•Extract maximum nutrition
•Eliminate dangerous foods.
•Achieve ideal body weight.
•Eat the right foods.

These are listed in progression. As you strive to achieve optimal health you will progress through the 4 levels. Everyone can do this. Let's start with number one.

Extract Maximum Nutrition

I never really understood the value of enzymes until I met Randy Grant. Randy has travelled all over the world and has served as nutritional consultant to Motorola, AT&T, NBA, NFL, Wesley Snipes, Arnold Schwarzenegger and countless others. Randy has seen it all when it comes to nutrition and diet trends. I was so impressed with Randy's resume I had him fly down from Arizona to my Fort Myers clinic so I could learn about his methods. About 10 minutes into his presentation Randy pulls out a Big Mac hamburger and sits it on the table. At the time, I was thinking maybe it was his lunch. He opens it up and asks me how it looked. There was no lettuce or tomatoes on it, just the white bread buns and 2 meat patties but it looked like a normal Big Mac. Here is what Randy tells me, he says the Big Mac is over 5 years old. First, I though wow that's great, it hasn't gone bad! Then I thought, why not? Randy says it is all about enzymes. Let me explain.

Enzymes are made inside the cells of living things and they are responsible for every action needed to maintain life. They are catalysts. Randy has a theory that humans have a predetermined amount of enzymes available and once the enzyme reserve is gone the person starts to degenerate. For example lactase is the enzyme needed to digest a protein found in milk, known as lactose. So once the person's reserve of lactase is used up they will not be able to digest milk any more and they become lactose intolerant. It is an interesting theory, one supported by notable physicians like, Dr. Hiromi Shinya, MD Chief Surgical Endoscopy of Beth Israel Medical Center. Dr. Hiromi states that by using specific enzyme therapies he has a 0% cancer recurrence rate. Let me repeat that in case you missed what I just wrote,

Dr. Hiromi states that his enzyme protocols have produced a 0% cancer recurrence rate. None have ever got sick with cancer again.

So the main idea is to not use up your body's enzyme reserve and it turns out that is easy to do because enzymes as exist in raw fruits and vegetables. So by eating a diet high in raw fruits and vegetables our body will use the enzymes provided in the food and not have to uses the ones we have stored in reserve. Enzymes are destroyed in temperatures above 118'F, which means that most any kind of prepared foods are enzyme deficient.

Initially the body may react to enzyme deficiency with what we call indigestion. Minor discomforts of burping, heartburn, abdominal cramping, pain and bad breath but more serious conditions like constipation, skin disorders, headaches and degenerative disease have also been linked to enzyme deficiency. There is something very ironic here in that when most people suffer from indigestion the first thing they reach for is an anti acid, which completely blocks the enzymes from doing there job. In most cases the person needs more enzymes and stomach acid not less.

So Randy is a big advocate of eating 50% raw fruits and vegetables every meal and taking digestive enzyme supplementation daily especially whenever your meal falls below the 50% mark. That way you are breaking down the foods you eat and preventing degenerative conditions like arthritis from developing. Randy has hundreds of testimonials from people who have completely changed there lives around just by taking a few digestive enzymes every time they eat. His evidence is so overwhelming that I personally carry digestive enzymes with me whenever I go out to eat, that way regardless of what food choices I am faced with the enzymes will make sure it causes the least amount of stress to my system.

I wish I could tell you that all you needed to do was eat fruit and vegetables to be healthy but that is not the case. Why? Well, it has a lot to do with growing conditions. Commercial growers over use the soil, so they must supplement with chemical to ensure a high yield. A non organic vegetable grown today contains less than 50% the nutritional content that it had just 100 years ago. So even someone doing everything right will need some level of enzyme support and of course if you are eating a high amount of cooked, processed foods it is critical to your health to supplement with digestive enzymes. So instead of running out and buying a multi vitamin why not eat better and take enzymes so your body can extract the nutrition out of the foods you eat? That is the first level of nutritional commitment I am asking you for. If nothing else take digestive enzymes with every meal, more if the food is processed less if you are having a raw salad.

The name of Randy's company is Divine Nature, I believe he is a great source for these products and information. I have bought enzymes from him and seen amazing results, both clinically and personally. I also like Optimal Health Systems, which incidentally is owned by Doug Grant, Randy's cousin. You will not be disappointed with either of these companies or their products. Here is a story about a patient of mine who accepted this first level of commitment and started taking Randy's digestive enzymes,

John was a construction worker who had suffered from heartburn that was getting worse. He was taking several prescriptions but losing the battle. His diet consisted of high fat, processed foods eaten on the run. Soda, beer, and milk were his favorite drinks. He was over weight, pre diabetic, high blood pressure, had a nasty, constant skin condition known as psoriasis and to top off the list suffered from moderate to severe back pain. He told me on the first visit he did not believe in Chiropractors and he wasn't going to change his diet. Or as he said he was not giving up his beer. I started him on digestive enzymes taken with each meal and started working on his back pain. Within 1 week he told me his heart burn was gone. By the end of the month his skin was clearing up, his blood sugar was coming down and his blood pressure had dropped so much that his prescribes medications had to be adjusted. I had his attention. John slowly started to follow my advice and the rest is history. His full testimonial is posted on my clinic wall. It all started with enzymes.

Vitamin and mineral requirements you should be getting,

Vitamin A - 5,000 IU
Beta carotene - 10,000 IU
Vitamin B-1 or thiamine - 1.5 mg
Vitamin B-2 or riboflavin - 1.7 mg
Niacin or niacin amide - 20 mg
Vitamin B-5 or pantothenic acid - 10 mg
Vitamin B-6 - 10 mg
Vitamin B-12 - 2.5 mcg.
Vitamin C - 250 mg
Vitamin D - 400 IU
Vitamin E - 200 IU
Vitamin K - 60 mcg
Folic Acid - 800 mcg
Biotin - 300 mcg

Calcium - 1,000 mg
Magnesium - 250 mg. Most people are magnesium deficient.
Iron - women 18 mg / men 10 mg.
Copper - 2 mg
Zinc - 15 mg
Selenium - 70 mcg
Chromium - 120 mcg
Iodine - 150 mcg
Manganese - 2 mg
Molybdenum -75 mcg
Boron - 3 mg
Silicon - 10 mg
Vanadium - 1 mg
Strontium - 1 mg
Cobalt - 25 mcg
Germanium - 100 mcg is a good dose.
Tin- 30 mcg
Nickel - 100 mcg
Rubidium - 1 mg
Cesium - 100 mcg

This is an exhaustive list of items so it just makes so much more sense to get these vitamins and minerals from the foods we eat by taking enzymes. Take 1-3 capsules depending on how much cooked or process food you are eating. If you take these with your meal it will help breakdown the food you are eating but if specific enzymes are taken on an empty stomach they can have a positive effect on helping overcome many common diseases like high cholesterol or high blood sugar. Enzymes are a new and exciting area of healthcare that I feel we will hear a lot more about in the future.

Eliminate Dangerous Foods

The next level to consider is getting rid of the really bad food choices that are directly related to disease and illness. I list them here for you consideration.

Carbonated Beverages

You may have to have Doctor Pepper now, and the fizzier the better, but later you will need Doctor Stokes. You have always heard that sodas are not good for you and you have heard how the caffeine, sugar, or the artificial sweetener is the problem. Well, there is another hidden problem that goes on inside a carbonated drink that you probably don't even know about and it is considered by most people to be the best part, the carbonation.

Our bodies are mostly made up of water. Water in a pure state has a neutral pH balance of 7. The values on the pH scale go from 0 to 14 with 0 being completely acidic and 14 being completely alkaline. That neutral level of 7 is where we want or bodies to be. The pH scale is exponential when a value drops a point. A 1 point drop on the pH scale is 10 times more acidic. For example, a drop from 7.0 to 6.0 is now 10 times more acidic than previously. From 7 to 5 is 100 times more acidic and so on. A rise in pH multiplies in the same way. Just like when the pH is out of balance on a swimming pool and bad algae begins to grow causing the pool to turn green, when we are out of proper pH, things that are not desirable can happen within us.

Carbonated beverages can greatly affect our pH level. When we talk about carbonation, we are not only talking about sodas. We also include sparkling water, sparkling ciders, and beer as well as others. The pH of regular and diet pops range from about 2.5 to 3.5 with the diet typically having a lower pH than the regular, sparkling waters are about 3-4, most beers are between 3.9 and 4.2, and ciders around 4.

In order to be at our healthiest, our pH should be somewhere from 7.1 to 7.5. Our blood should be from 7.35 to 7.45. Just about everything we do moves us towards a more acidic pH. Most of the foods we consume are digested down to acids. We also create acids throughout our body when we exercise. Diseases definitely thrive in acidic, oxygen poor environments and carbonated beverages assist the creation of more acid.

When the terminal of a car battery is covered with corrosion from sulfuric acid in the battery attacking the lead post, we can neutralize the buildup by pouring carbonated liquid over the acid buildup. When we ingest food our stomach produces hydrochloric acid (HCl) to begin the digestive process. Unfortunately when we drink carbonated liquids (carbonic acid), with our food we neutralizing the HCl. By neutralizing the HCl, we send an internal message to our pancreas not to send enzymes to aid in the digestion of the food, thus allowing the food to sit in our stomach undigested. By drinking a soda with a meal, even the most balanced, healthy menu can be sabotaged because nutrients in the food are not digested and absorbed. It can't pass through and be put to its proper use.

Your body will try to protect you as long as it can compensate. When you drink a carbonated beverage, the body will use reserves of its own stored alkaline buffers, mainly calcium from the bones and DNA to raise the body's alkalinity level, to maintain a proper pH level, especially the pH of the blood. When your kidneys are overtaxed from trying to buffer the intake of acid foods and beverages that the body can't compensate fully, the problems begin. Kidney and gall stones can form, joint pain can result from the crystallizing deposits, the vascular system becomes calcified and narrows caused by hardening and blocking of the arteries. Carbonated drinks have also been shown to contribute to osteoporosis and dental erosion. Without enough minerals to go around, muscle spasms are common. Sleep and relaxation may not be regular. Damage to cells, free radicals, as a result of out of balance pH in the blood, can be seen under a microscope.

Will we die from drinking carbonated beverages? If your body could not neutralize these acids, you would die. Every carbonated beverage you drink raises your acidity and speeds up the aging process. If you must have a carbonated beverage, have it as a between meal snack but best would be to reach for the water, fruit or vegetable juice, or green tea. If you want to help your body's natural process of reducing acid preform this one time treatment to balance your pH,

Juice 10 whole lemons and put into 3 quarts water. Drink slowly over 24 hours. Lemon can balance the body by raising or lowering pH as needed.

Milk - Natures Perfect Food (NO!)

Everyone is familiar with milk and it's related dairy products. I was raised on milk. During high school when I was trying to gain weight for Rugby, I drank 2 liters of whole milk everyday. I though milk was a health food loaded with calories and protein and it sure packed on the pounds. I remember reading in my college nutrition book that milk is natures perfect food. What I did not realize then, was that like all processed foods, milk was not good for my body. Before processing, milk contains many good elements however it loses all these good qualities to manufacturing. Here is the process. First the suction machine is attached to the cows nipple squeezing out the milk which is then stored temporarily in a tank. The raw milk collected at each farmhouse is then transferred into an even bigger tank and is stirred and homogenized. This is a process that prevents the fat in milk from separating and rising to the top. It changes the fat in milk to hydrogenated fat which is the bad fat. Now before going to market homogenized milk must be heat pasteurized to suppress the propagation of various germs and bacteria. This is done using sustained high temperature. Because enzymes are sensitive to heat they breakdown and are completely lost. Remember, enzymes are of vital importance fro every body function and prevention of disease. Also at the ultrahigh temperatures used in pasteurization more hydrogenated fat is created. So the processing of milk kills all the good enzymes and transforms the fat found in milk into a poison.

There is a big misconception that milk helps prevent osteoporosis. Not true. Drinking too much milk will cause osteoporosis, here's how. The calcium concentration in human blood is normally fixed at 9 to 10 mg however when you drink milk the calcium concentration of your blood suddenly rises. When this happens the body tries to bring this level back to normal by excreting calcium from the kidney. So if you try to drink milk, to get calcium, this process produces the ironic result of decreasing the overall level of calcium in the body. All the big four dairy countries America, Sweden, Denmark and Finland, where a lot of milk is consumed every day, have high occurrences of hip fractures and osteoporosis. In contrast to this countries like Japan, where people consume many small fish, containing calcium that is not quickly absorbed in a way that raises the blood calcium concentration level have very low rates of bone loss diseases like osteoporosis. If you can find unpasteurized organic milk from grass fed cows these problems do not apply but then you have to consider the potential of germs and disease being transferred from the cow into your body. Most unpasteurized milk cannot be sold for human consumption because of this problem. Of course if you live near a farm that you are comfortable with you will be able to enjoy clean, organic, unpasteurized milk. Otherwise take a pass.

Grains

Grain consumption is a sensitive subject for many individuals, so I want to spend some time explaining why I feel it is not a good food choice. Most people have eaten bread, pasta, and cereals their entire lives, and giving up this food can be psychologically traumatic for some, which illustrates the strong and often inappropriate emotional connection that we have with food. Many find it surprising that grains are a relatively new food from a historical perspective.

The following foods were never consumed before 5,000-10,000 years ago: grains, pasta, cereal, soy, beans, dairy, refined sugar, partially hydrogenated fats, and seed oils, such as corn, safflower, cottonseed, sunflower, peanut, canola, and soybean oil.

Mammals with a similar genetic code to ours inhabited the earth for 1,990,000 years before man appeared on earth. We must appreciate that our genes are not dissimilar from those that came before us; modern science has demonstrated this fact. This means that humans are genetically adapted to eat fruits, vegetables, fish, fowl, meat, roots, tubers, and nuts. Consider also that there are no chronic diseases caused by eating these foods. No matter what disease you may suffer from, none of these foods must be eliminated from the diet. The same cannot be said for grains. In a nutshell, grains contain several problematic substances including gluten, lectin, and phytates. Grains also promote inflammation by increasing body acidity, and disrupting proper blood sugar regulation. I have experimented with many different diets and tested the blood chemistry of patients both on and off grains. In every case elimination of grains promoted health. This research even changed my own dietary choices and moved me from the vegetarian diet I had followed for many years to my current diet that does not include many grains.

Gluten

Celiac disease is a disabling digestive condition that is caused by the gluten found in certain grains. Most notorious on the list of gluten grains is wheat; others include couscous, spelt, kamut, rye, and barley. Among the non-gluten grains are rice, wild rice, millet, and corn. You may be familiar with Celiac disease which is a condition that damages the lining of the small intestine and prevents it from absorbing parts of food that are important for staying healthy. The damage is due to a reaction to eating gluten, which is found in wheat, barley, rye, and possibly oats. The exact cause of celiac disease is unknown. The lining of the intestines contains areas called villi, which help absorb nutrients. When people with celiac disease eat foods or use products that contain gluten, their immune system reacts by damaging these villi. This damage affects the ability to absorb nutrients properly. A person becomes malnourished no matter how much food he or she eats. The disease can develop at any point in life, from infancy to late adulthood. People who have a family member with celiac disease are at greater risk for developing the disease. The disorder is most common in Caucasians and persons of European ancestry. Women are affected more often than men. Here is the big point you need to understand,

It is not only those suffering from celiac disease that need to avoid grains. Gluten can promote many other symptoms and conditions, ranging from schizophrenia to more common conditions such as headaches. For certain individuals, gluten sensitivity can present exclusively as a neurologic disease, and not with classic digestive problems. The most common symptoms include headache and nervous system symptoms such as numbness, tingling, and weakness.

In one study researchers randomly selected 200 disease-free individuals for the purpose of assessing anti-gluten antibody levels, which is a way to measure gluten sensitivity. Health complaints of the 15% of subjects with the highest antibody levels were compared with the 15% of subjects with the lowest levels.

Interestingly, those with the highest antibody levels suffered from headaches, chronic fatigue, regular digestive complaints, subtle anemic changes, and NO signs of celiac disease, while those with the lowest levels were symptom-free. In another report, 3 cases of gluten sensitivity were discussed. All patients were women in their mid 40's and each suffered from digestive bloating, gas, abdominal pain, and fatigue. Symptoms resolved after going on gluten-free diet. A detailed list of gluten foods can be found at the Celiac Sprue Association's website (www.csaceliacs.org). Here is a personal story about my wife's struggle with gluten.

Kathy (my wife) developed a strange problem several years ago where every time she tried to write with her left hand the index finger would curled up. After I ran all my tests, I was still undecided. I brought her to several specialists and we did some brain scans. The diagnosis was early onset of Parkinson's. Wow. That was a real eye opener. I took Kathy to a neurologist in Naples that specialized in neurological disorders and after extensive testing he looked at me and said your wife does not have Parkinson's disease, it is just a dystonia. Great, I though. Now what? The outcome was that nothing I did helped her dystonia until one day after being on a high protein diet for about 7 days (no grains!) Kathy was signing a credit card receipt and stopped. She looked over at me, no more curled finger. Cured. Amazing. By removing the gluten from her diet she repaired her condition. I hate to say this but later when she returned to a normal diet that included pasta, her dystonia came back. These are hard lessons to learn. The interesting thing about Kathy's condition was that I tested her for gluten sensitivity and the results were negative. Still by reducing her intake of grains and sugar her disorder got better. So just because your doctor tells you that you do not have a gluten sensitivity does not mean you will not benefit from reducing grains.

Grains contain a substance called phytic acid, which is known to reduce the absorption of calcium, magnesium and zinc. Grains also promote an acidic body pH, which is known to

5' 0"	97 -- 128	108 -- 138
5'1"	101 -- 132	111 -- 143
5'2"	14 -- 137	115 -- 148
5'3"	107 -- 141	119 -- 152
5'4"	111 -- 146	122 -- 157
5'5"	114 -- 150	126 -- 162
5'6"	118 -- 155	130 -- 167
5'7"	121 -- 160	134 -- 172
5'8"	125 -- 164	138 -- 178
5'9"	129 -- 169	142 -- 183
5'10"	132 -- 174	146 -- 188
5"11"	136 -- 179	151 -- 194
6'0"	140 -- 184	155 -- 199
6'1"	144 -- 189	159 -- 205
6'2"	148 -- 195	164 -- 210
6'3"	152 -- 200	168 -- 216
6'4"	156 -- 205	173 -- 222
6'5"	160 -- 211	177 -- 228

be inflammatory. Research has now demonstrated that a diet induced acidic state helps to promote the loss of bone and muscle. While grains are a low-fat food, they contain an elevated ratio of omega-6 to omega-3 fatty acids. Omega-6 fatty acids are converted into chemicals the cause inflammation, chronic disease, and pain. So benefit is outweighed by the problems.

With the above in mind, you may be wondering why we have been told that grains are so good for us? First, whole grains do contain nutrients and fiber, both of which are healthy and anti-inflammatory. However, we get more nutrients and fiber from fruits and vegetables. Second, grains are inexpensive and can be stored easily, so they are profitable for food manufacturers. We are never told that we can get all the nutrients and fiber we require by eating fruits, vegetables, and nuts, and that there is no need to consume grains. It is important to understand that the health conditions discussed above have only been associated with the consumption of grains and legumes (beans) and have never ever been associated with the consumption of fruits, vegetables, nuts, and healthy animal meats. Therefore, try to avoid grains, flours, bread, pasta, etc., and try to replace these foods with fruits and vegetables.

What About Fiber?

A great misconception is the notion that we cannot get adequate fiber unless we eat whole grains. In fact, whole grains are a poor source of fiber when compared to fruits and vegetables on a calorie basis. When we compare foods based on calories, fresh fruit typically contains twice the amount of fiber found in whole grains, and non-starchy vegetables, such as broccoli and lettuce, contain almost 8 times the amount of fiber found in whole grains.

Along with being low in fiber, grains are also low in potassium when compared to fruits and vegetables. Research has demonstrated that diets low in potassium predispose one to numerous diseases such as chronic pain, osteoporosis, age related muscle wasting, calcium kidney stones, high blood pressure, stroke, asthma, exercise-induced asthma, insomnia, air sickness, high-altitude sickness, Meniere's Syndrome (ear ringing), and age and disease related chronic kidney insufficiency.

Unlike other minerals, it is important that we get potassium from food, not supplements. Supplementing with potassium can lead to inappropriately high levels of potassium in the blood, called hyperkalemia, which can lead to muscle weakness, numbness and tingling, abnormal heart rhythm, muscle paralysis, troubled breathing, and even heart failure and death.

Lectins

All grains and legumes (beans, lentils, soy) also contain sugar proteins called lectins, which resist digestion and cooking. Before absorption, lectins are known to cause digestive system inflammation, which may or may not cause obviously linked symptoms. After lectins are absorbed into circulation from the digestive tract, they bind the surface of cells throughout the body. While all the details are not known, researchers state that,

There is now abundant evidence that lectins can cause disease in man and animals.

I believe lectins play a role in promoting the following conditions,

- Inflammatory bowel disease
- Diabetes mellitus
- Rheumatoid arthritis
- Psoriasis
- Multiple sclerosis
- Retinitis and cataracts
- Congenital malformations
- Infertility
- Allergies and other autoimmune problems

Just the fact that beans need to be prepared so much before we can eat them should be an obvious sign that they are not an ideal food source for humans.

Artificial Sweeteners

Everybody loves sugar but your body knows the difference between sugar and artificial sweeteners. Sugar is sucrose, fructose and maltose, that's it. Check the labels because every few years a new artificial sweetener is introduced that is guaranteed to be safe, every one of these artificial non-caloric sweeteners has been found to be toxic and unsafe. One of the most popular products is Splenda. It is advertised that it tastes like sugar and is made from sugar. This is a lie, this is not true. Splenda is a chemically modified substance where chlorine is added to the chemical structure, making it more similar to a chlorinated pesticide than something we should be eating or drinking. As this breaks down in your body it creates more unnatural products that helps to destroy your digestive system. Most people think that they are doing something good for themselves by choosing the "diet" drinks or "lite" yogurts compared to the sugar-laden versions, but the problem is that you're exposing yourself to a whole new set of problems with the artificially sweetened drinks and foods. Always choose sugar over artificial sweeteners.

Another product I hear a lot about in the media is Stevia. This seems good at first because it is a plant and not made in a lab. Unfortunately natural does not always mean safe. As an example tobacco is also natural plant. The FDA has refused to approve the entire plant extract as a sugar substitute. All the studies show that Stevia, Sucralose, Aspartame, and all sugar substitutes do the same if not more damage than regular sugar. So why bother? If you must use sugar, read labels and look for sugar or better yet look for products without sugar. Enough said.

Achieve Ideal Body Weight

When it comes down to maintaining body weight it is all about how many calories you consume. I wish it was not. I wish we could lose weight by just eating healthy, but you will gain weight if you eat healthy, too often. The first thing we need to do is evaluate your current body weight. Using the chart find out where you stand right now. This will give you goals and guidelines to follow. Low numbers are generally assigned to women, high numbers to men. If you are more than 20 pounds overweight you will need drastic changes in your lifestyle to make any progress. It is my suggestion patients who are severely over weight fast. In my experience with thousands of overweight patients it is just not possible to make the types of changes necessary by following a normal healthy food plan. We have to get the extra weight off and we need to eliminate all that extra fat. Fat acts like a gland and secretes chemicals that causes pain and degenerative diseases.

Fasting is easy to do. Just stop eating. BUT NEVER STOP DRINKING WATER. The goal is to flip your body over into ketosis within the first 3 days on the fast. You can buy ketone test strips at the drug store and check yourself each day. If after the third day you do not get into ketosis YOU MUST STOP THE FAST. This is very serious and very important. In a small number of people they are not able to convert over into ketosis. If you don't convert you will starve yourself and your body will begin to break down until it finally dies. If you convert into ketosis than you will not starve, instead your body will breakdown all the extra fat and material that it is carrying and burn it as fuel. You will literally eat up or burn off all the extra fat and weight without losing muscle. Sounds easy? Anyone who tells me that has never fasted. It is hard and the first 3 days are the hardest because your body will still be using glucose as fuel so you will feel tired and sickly. Once you hit ketosis you will drop 2 pounds a day, some patients drop even more. Again, you must drink lots of fluid during the fast. Food, you can live without but you cannot live without water.

I have personally fasted for 14 consecutive days. During my fast I lost about 20 pounds. It completely got rid of my love handles and I felt great. When you break a fast you must slowly ease back into eating solid foods again or you will get sick. I like to start with broths and work up to steamed veggies and eventually eat some broiled white fish. Once you hit your weight goal then you can begin to follow the guidelines presented here on eating the right amount and correct type of foods to keep you at that weight level. If I have a patient that needs to lose, 50-100 pounds, I will usually fast them for a week, lose 10 pounds, stabilize them for a few weeks then fast them again, perhaps this time for 2 weeks and continue in this stepping manner until I get all the weight off.

Now for some confessions. Fasting is hard. I will usually drink coffee, black tea or green tea several times a day to maintain energy levels. Yes, this is bad. Yes, this can be very dangerous because it can dehydrate you, so you MUST MAINTAIN HIGH FLUID LEVELS DURING A FAST. I have experimented with a small bit of almond milk in the coffee and so far it has not broken my ketosis. You can check with the ketone strips. Like I said, I know coffee is bad. I get it. But you are going to be hungry, your body may need a stimulant unless you plan on just resting at home for the next week. Coffee is bad but the extra fat on your body is much worse. If this does not make sense to you, don't do it. I am just telling you how I get through it. You will never change without drastic steps. As I write this chapter I am in the middle of a week long fast (not planned, weird huh?) I started at 192 lb. and today, 6 days in, I am 184 lb. Last night I ate 3 fresh gulf shrimp because I felt weak. Never hurt anything and I am back on track today, working in my study, writing this book and sipping Earl Grey tea. That is reality.

Exercise is a big no-no while fasting. Do as little as possible. Also depending on a patients health condition I may have them load up on digestive enzymes during the fast that are designed to breakdown fats and sugars. Since you are not eating the enzymes are used by the body to help the weight loss and clean out the system.

Fasting is nothing new. It has been around for hundreds of years. I fast one week every year and one day every week. It is a great way to stay in touch with your body. Remember dynamic effort is needed for real life changing results. Just do it. I would like to again refer you to Dr. Joel Furhman's book if you are serious about fasting. He covers information about hypoglycemia and other myths about fasting.

Let's say you are at your ideal weight and want to stay there, no problem, but you are going to have to understand calories and how they are transferred into body weight. Here is a lesson.

Each pound of body weight will need between 10 (inactive) to 15 (athlete) calories to maintain. So lets assume a person weights 200 pounds. They will need to take in 200 x 10 = 2000 calories a day just to maintain that weight.

When someone is overweight and tells me they only eat salads I know they are lying. Unless they are eating salads with a gallon of blue cheese dressing. I know this is a touchy subject but we have to be honest with each other if we are going to make a change and these numbers do not lie. This is based on a weekly intake of food not an isolated day or 2 of light eating. Let me give an example here so I can win you onside.

I saw this little girl that was overweight and needing my help, she was about 10 years old. When I asked about diet I was told by her parents she only ate small healthy meals. I calculated the numbers and told them, no way. They got mad with me and I had to bring in a nurse to speak with them because they thought I was making stuff up. Anyways, we all came to find out the little girl is drinking 5-6 sodas a day. BINGO! Enough said. I can tell anyone how much they eat on average each day if they tell me their weight. It is just math.

Each pound of body fat contains about 3500 calories. So if you cut your daily intake by 500 calories (500 calories/ day x 7 days = 3500 calories), you will lose 1 pound a week.

Not a lot. Like I said, fasting is a better way to reduce body weight. Once you have reached your ideal body weight maintain it with the right amount of calories and the right types of food.

Eat The Correct Foods

Usually when patients come into my clinic they are ready to experience something different. They may have heard from other patients about some unique procedure we do or how we test the blood in a special way or just that we treat the most difficult cases. So they have high expectations from the start. They hang on every word I say and look at me like I am some sort of magician that is going to just wave a wand and presto, all is better. Then comes, what I refer to as, the first reality check. I tell them as part of my program they will receive the most powerful medicine available, so strong that if they did nothing else the results would be extraordinary. "Yes doctor", they say nodding their heads, "Yes, whatever you recommend I will do". Then I say to them, "The most powerful medicine is your diet." Everything goes silent. Some roll their eyes, some stare blankly and some just keep nodding waiting for me to deliver the promised information despite the fact that I already have just told them. Diet. Nasty word isn't it. Over rated, over promoted and definitely represents some sort of failure for most people. Bad news is that you cannot get away from it. Not in my office. Sorry and here's the real rub, when I say diet, I don't just mean losing some weight and cutting back on sweets. When I say diet I mean complete lifestyle modification. If this sounds intense, that's because it is.

There is a very good chance everything you are currently eating is wrong and all your ideas about nutrition are wrong. It is interesting that I get more opposition on my diet recommendations than anything else. I do procedures in my office that cost thousands of dollars and patients never question them, but the diet stuff, which is free, they will fight me on. Go figure! Food is everything and food is everywhere. What you eat combined with your specific genetics is directly responsible for the state of your health. After 10 years of researching food and it's relationship to human disease, I'm convinced that the ideal diet is one consisting mostly of vegetables and lean proteins with a limited intake of fruit. Before I give you the ideal eating plan here are 5 points to always keep in mind whenever you are thinking about nutrition.

1. The whole is greater than the sum of its parts.

2. Genes do not determine disease on their own. Genes function only by being activated, or expressed, and nutrition plays a critical role in determining which genes, good or bad, are expressed.

3. Nutrition can substantially control the adverse effects of toxic chemical exposure.

4. The same nutrition that prevents disease in its early stages (before diagnosis) can also halt or reverse disease in its later stages (after diagnosis).

5. Nutrition that is truly beneficial for one chronic disease will support health across the board. This is a point that makes everything so easy, don't you agree?

You need to make a choice regarding the foods you eat: will they be disease promoting foods or healing foods? If you feel great and do not have any health problems you still need to consider the risk of regularly consuming bad foods that are known to cause significant health problems and disease. Within a week of starting to eat this way you are likely to experience a difference in how you feel. After 1 month you will know for sure how food affects your health (some people who are significantly sick may need 2-3 months). The focus of my dietary recommendations is reducing inflammation and chronic disease. We all have a problem with inflammation to some degree and in many cases people just do not know how sick they are until they get better. Does that make sense? If not maybe it will once you start eating the right foods.

How Diet Relates To Pain

Doctors are usually focused on structural diagnosis and they forget that pain is never just mechanical. To experience pain you must have a chemical reaction. Inflammation is the main trigger that ignites pain. Inflammation needs to occur after an injury takes place and it is an important part of healing however when chronic inflammation takes place we see a promotion of diseases like cancer, hypertension and heart disease. Even Alzheimer disease, osteoarthritis, rheumatoid arthritis, diabetes and even menopause can develop and continue to exist as a consequence of chronic inflammation.

Humans are genetically programmed to eat a diet that is mostly anti-inflammatory. This consists mainly of vegetables, fruits, nuts and animals that eat vegetation. This is commonly known as a hunter or Paleolithic diet. In contrast today's modern diet is based largely on grains and animals that eat grains. In addition there are many refined foods like sodas and engineered foods. This modern diet promotes inflammation and the main metabolic imbalance that promotes disease, insulin resistance.

Insulin Resistance

We breakdown carbohydrates into glucose so our cells can use them as energy. Insulin is a special chemical that we use to allow this to occur. If our carbohydrate load becomes excessive more insulin is needed and eventually our cells become less responsive to allowing the glucose into the cells. The glucose cannot remain in the blood so it is then forced to be stored in our fat cells. Eventually these inflated fat cells begin excreting hormones that cause many health problems. Just think of all the sugar soda pop people are drinking today, this along is responsible for the wide increase in insulin resistance and subsequently diabetes in todays younger population.

Contrary to popular belief fats (monounsaturated fatty acids) found in nuts, olive oil and animal products can promote insulin sensitivity and actually lower inflammation. A high carbohydrate low fat diet would be the worse choice for anyone trying to fight disease. This type of eating will make you sick.

Foods To Avoid

- Grains and grain products, including white bread, whole wheat bread, pasta, cereal, pretzels, crackers, and any other product made with grains or flours from grains, which includes most desserts and packaged snacks.

- Partially hydrogenated oils trans fats) found in margarine, deep fried foods (French fries, etc.) and most all packaged foods.

- Corn oil, safflower oil, sunflower oil, cottonseed oil, peanut oil, soybean oil, and foods made with these oils such as mayonnaise, tartar sauce, margarine, salad dressings, and many packaged foods.

- Soda and sugar are inflammatory. If you eat dairy or soy, they should be consumed as condiments, not staples.

- Meat and eggs from grain-fed animals (domesticated animal products). Modern meat is problematic because the animals are obese and unhealthy; they are loaded with saturated fats and contain too many pro-inflammatory omega-6 fatty acids. Grass-fed meat or wild game are our best choices. Otherwise, we should eat lean meat, skinless chicken, omega-3 eggs and wild fish. Lean cuts of meat and lean hamburger meat are available at most grocery stores, and even extra-lean is sometimes available.

I know that it can seem over whelming and you may feel that there is nothing left to eat, however, you need to decide how much pain and suffering you are willing to live with, and then, eat accordingly. The fewer inflammatory foods you eat, the less inflammation you will have and feel. No one will be perfect with their eating, just do your best. If you have a few weak moments or longer periods of time where you dine excessively on inflammatory foods, do not beat yourself up or become depressed. This happens to everyone, so simply recommit yourself to the program. Stay focused and tell your self that every thing you consume will take you one step closer to health or disease. This is a fact we all must accept, so we should all do our best to make good choices.

If you are fortunate and have "good" genes, you may be able to handle more inflammatory foods than some of your family members or friends. The problem is that most inflammatory diseases develop slowly and without symptoms until it is far too late. Therefore, we all need to be careful about consuming pro inflammatory foods and not take for granted what appears to be good health.

All you need to do is eat mostly fruits, vegetables, nuts, fish, chicken, and lean meat. Eat until you begin to feel full and then stop. Occasionally I will place patients on complete vegetable diets but I have found over the years this is not necessary for most people. As I gather practical research from my own patients, I feel that the complete absence of animal products is not necessary. Recently, I am seeing more problems with a strict vegetarian diet that promotes many grains and grain products.

Foods That Promote Health

- All fruits and vegetables. Eat fruits raw and vegetables raw or lightly cooked.

- Red and sweet potatoes are acceptable as long as they are consumed with a protein, such as eggs, fish, meat, or fowl.

- Fresh or frozen fish. This must be wild. Farm raised fish has high levels of omega-6 fatty acids.

- Meat, chicken, eggs from grass-fed animals. Go to www.eatwild.com to find producers of grass-fed animal products. If you cannot acquire grass-fed products, do the best you can to get lean cuts of regular meats, which are available at all supermarkets.

- Omega-3 eggs. There is usually local farm raised eggs available from cage free animals. You will notice the difference in taste and the color of the yolk, it is brilliant yellow.

- Wild game (deer, elk, etc.) Here in Florida it is easy to get wild boar.

- Nuts: raw almonds, cashews, walnuts, hazelnuts, macadamia nuts, etc. As nuts are high in calories, be sure to temper your nut consumption if your goal is to lose weight. For example, 1/4 cup of nuts provides about 170-225 calories. Try to buy raw nuts, once they are roasted and salted they are just junk food. The roasting process destroys the oils (hydrogenates).

- Spices like ginger, turmeric, garlic, dill, oregano, fennel, red chili pepper (my favorite), basil, rosemary, and even a little sea salt is okay.

- Oils and fats: It is best to use organic oils, as it is thought that non-organic oils may contain pesticides. Use organic extra virgin olive oil and coconut oil. Butter is also a healthy choice and the best butter comes from grass fed cows. You will get the best available butter if you buy organic butter (Organic Valley indicates that their butter and heavy cream are from grass-fed cows).

- Salad dressing: extra virgin olive oil, balsamic vinegar (or lemon juice), mustard if you like, and spices (Greek, Italian, ginger, dill, oregano, etc.; whatever suits your taste). When eating in a restaurant, use dressings sparingly, as most are made with soybean oil or worse, and most are rich in sugar.

- Whenever you are thirsty, drink water or organic green tea (non-organic tea may contain pesticides and should be avoided).

- Instead of rice, pasta or other grain product, have more vegetables and a modest potato portion with whatever protein dish is being served.

Breakfast Options

Breakfast is very important, try not to miss it. Include some of these food selections.

- Soft boiled, poached or gently fried omega-3 eggs and favorite vegetables and spices (a small serving of sautéed potatoes is okay if you are not carbohydrate sensitive). It is best to use organic virgin coconut oil for cooking eggs and potatoes. Olive oil would be the next best option.

- Omega-3 egg or egg white omelet with favorite vegetables and spices. You can pour marinara or pasta sauce over the omelet. When you add the sauce, it tastes like a pizza.

- Oatmeal or grits. To avoid excess calories, use water instead of milk [or soy/rice/ almond milk] and let the fruit be your sweetener.

- Favorite fruit topped with a quarter cup of your favorite nut that has been previously soaked in water. Blend the soaked nut with water and pour over the fruit.

Lunch and Dinner Options

- A chicken, fish, or steak Caesar salad without croutons is an example of a meal that contains appropriate portions of vegetables and protein; it is a model meal that can be applied to all other meals when determining your vegetable and protein portions.

- Chicken, fish, steak (or favorite lean meat) and steamed/ sautéed vegetables with favorite spices. You can have a small portion of sautéed or baked potato. Have as much salad as you like.

- Marinara or pasta sauce poured over vegetables and meatballs from lean chop meat (or animal protein sources of your choice).

- Have as much salad as you like with lunch and dinner

When you feel like you have room for dessert, eat more vegetables, or wait an hour to see if you are indeed still hungry, and don't forget to take your enzymes.

Meal Shake

Since everyone is in a hurry these days, including me, I find that often I will have a meal shake. You can blend your favorite frozen fruit (bananas, blueberries, cherries, strawberries, etc.) and egg white protein powder (or protein powder of choice). You can also add some coconut or your favorite raw nut. Make sure to always use water for blending to avoid excess calories. This shake is not only highly nutritious and filling, but easy and quick to prepare. Avoid products with artificial sweeteners or vitamins and minerals, just get the simple proteins. Go to the local body building nutrition shop and ask about high quality protein powders, just make sure not to use anything with artificial sweeteners. I have been seen at the Smoothie King buying a Gladiator.

Snack Options

- Any combination of your favorite fresh fruits. 1-2 Tbsp of organic heavy cream over frozen cherries, blueberries, or favorite fruit. I know this is dairy, I know but we are talking 2 tablespoons, a far cry, from an ice cream banana split.

- Dark chocolate, raisins, and raw almonds or favorite raw nut. Again nuts are high in calories, so be sure to temper your nut consumption if your goal is to lose weight. For example, 1/4 cup of nuts provides about 170-240 calories. When eating dark chocolate, try to use 50 calorie pieces, as chocolate is also high in calories.

Please realize that you may not have to significantly alter the meals you currently prepare. Simply substitute vegetables for grains, bread, and pasta, and eat more fruit (or healthy dessert/ snack options) between meals. Clearly, there is no need to make healthy eating a complicated or negative process. In general, make your lunch and dinner choices of eggs, meat, fish, and chicken fit in the 25% protein section of the meal plate. The remaining 75% of the plate should be piled high with vegetables. It cannot be much simpler, just buy the highest quality foods you can afford.

Summary

1. Extract Maximum Nutrition

- Take Digestive Enzymes With Every Meal

2. Eliminate Dangerous Foods

-Avoid carbonated drinks, processed milk, grains and grain products, lectins and artificial sweeteners

3. Achieve Ideal Body Weight.

-Use cyclic fasting to achieve goal weight then calorie counting to maintain it.

4. Eat the right foods.

-Anti-inflammatory diet of natural foods.

Step Six: Activate Mitochondria

And now for something completely different.
-Monty Python's Flying Circus
(Just seeing if you are paying attention)

Cellular Energy

You have little batteries inside of your cells and they are called the Mitochondria. These entities things once lived outside of our system and a long time ago decided to join our cells for a mutually beneficial relationship. These parts of our cells are so amazing I am including here a brief explanation of how this happened from one of the smartest, up and coming scientists I know, Michael McDowell. Mike is currently attending St. Louis University on full scholarship. He frequently scores grades on his exams of 100%. That's right 100%. He claims that he wants to go to medical school but I think that would be a waste of his potential. The world would benefit much more

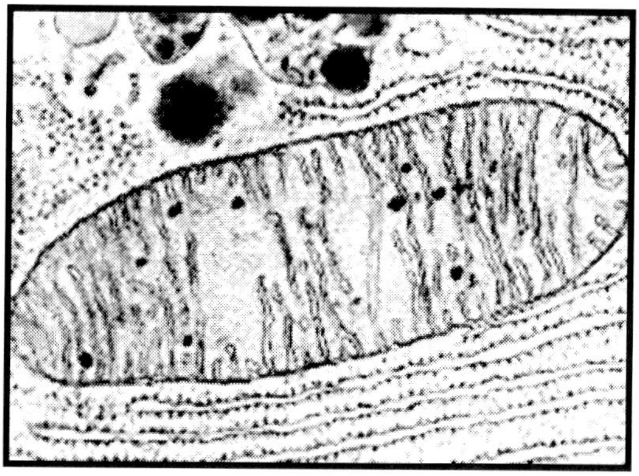

if he went into full time research. Of course Mike is my step son and he just happens to hold a passion for Mitochondria. I asked him to write this brief explanation of why the Mitochondria are so important.

The Endosymbiotic Theory stems from all of the indications that we know of both the structure and function of Mitochondria. Primarily, Mitochondria possess a double membrane in which the processes of cellular respiration uses oxygen and components that are broken down from the food we ingest to produce ATP, the basis for all cellular energy. This double membrane is thought to have formed from an event in which the Mitochondria, acting as a lone prokaryotic cell, was actually engulfed by another cell that would eventually lead to the creation of the cells present in our body. This engulfment created the secondary membrane that surrounds the mitochondria.

Another indication that Mitochondria once existed as a lone entity is that they possess their own DNA. The Mitochondria's DNA is present in a circular form and ours is the familiar double helix. Overtime however, much of the DNA needed for the function of Mitochondria seems to have been transferred to the nucleus of our cells making the Mitochondria dependent on the coding found in our DNA for their survival and function.

Basically what all of this indicates is that a long time ago, cells that would eventually make up the multicellular organization found in the human body existed independently. These cells, only being able to produce small amounts of energy through an anaerobic (without oxygen) processing of organic material, came upon mitochondria, like bacterium, that could be harnessed to more efficiently produce energy through an aerobic process (using oxygen). These cells then engulfed or ate these bacteria and eventually made them dependent. In a sense the mitochondria were made slaves to produce large amounts of energy for the cell that allowed them to form multicellular organism like human beings.

Interesting Point: The DNA of the Mitochondria and common bacteria are very similar. I believe it is possible that extensive

use of prescription antibiotics can collaterally damage the Mitochondria when attacking the harmful bacteria. This could lead to premature aging, less energy and degenerative disease. Antibiotic therapy should be closely monitored. This is only a theory of mine but based on my research it certainly makes sense.
-Mike McDowell

The Mitochondria produce a molecule called ATP, Adenosine Triphosphate which is the basic energy source of your entire body. A healthy Mitochondria produces about 1% waste from this process of making ATP and the exhaust comes in the form of free radicals. These are molecules that have an unpaired electron in the outer orbit. This makes them very unstable and highly reactive. The unpaired electron is always trying to stabilize itself by reacting with other molecules that can donate an electron. This exchange produces inflammation and damages our cellular structures. When the production of ATP becomes less effective the waste produced increases. Think of this like someone reaching their anaerobic threshold while they are working out, lactic acid builds up, they get tired and the muscles start to ache. These free radicals lead to aging and disease and eventually when we produce more waste than can be processed we die. Keeping this system working at optimal capacity is very important. The biggest threats are toxins. These include poisons from environmental exposure (pesticides, radiation, second hand smoke) and from the foods we eat (sugar, additives, hydrogenated oils).

Our bodies produce a safety mechanism for handling free radical activity called antioxidants. These are substances like vitamin C and can be found in many fruits and vegetables we eat. Glutathione is one of the most powerful antioxidants available and should be included in any health building program. A excellent teacher of mine, Dr. Walter H. Schmittt, once commented,

Antioxidants are like bullet proof vests for our cells.

The good doctor really helped me understand the benefits of these powerful chemicals. It is directly because of his teachings that I started to change my own diet and regulate the foods I eat. Recently, there have been several studies that show a restrictive caloric intake reduces free radical activity. Another good reason for periodic fasting and lot's of fruits and vegetables. I want to tell you a true story about a past patient of mine that shows how important anti oxidants can be...

Donald Lasko was diagnosed with cancer when he came into my office. I told Don, I don't treat cancer and he said I don't care just do whatever you can to help me fight this thing. At the time I was doing very little nutrition. I started adjusting his body to free him of Subluxations. There have been several valid studies that report chiropractic manipulation can increase your immune system activity. Either way I thought he would be better off if he was free from joint fixation. During the time he was my patient he started taking huge dosages of vitamin C. He had read some articles by Linus Pauling.

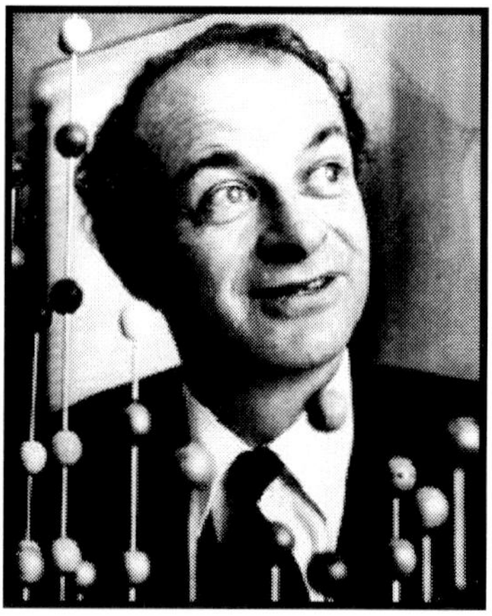

Pauling is one of only four individuals to have won more than one Nobel Prize. He had strong ideas about the use antioxidants. and was a brilliant chemist. So based on Pauling's teachings Don was taking somewhere around 15,000 mg of vitamin C a day, that's 15 grams! In about 4 weeks his blood chemistry started to change and his cancer doctor told him that his blood cell count had gone way down. This continued and eventually Don was given the great news that he was cancer free. Amazing. The cancer doctor at first thought it was the crazy chiropractor who recommended all that vitamin C but no I had nothing to do with it. Just think of what could be possible if this type of knowledge could find it's way into main stream medicine. Linus Pauline and his teachings are the foundation of what is now called orthomolecular medicine, or functional medicine.

Remember these stories when someone tells you there is nothing that can be done. It usually means you just need to look a little harder. Also remember what my step son, Michael McDowell mentioned about how antibiotics may be injuring the Mitochondria. Don't abuse these powerful drugs and increase your probiotic intake after using antibiotics to help reestablish your gut flora. Antibiotic use may have a strong correlation to Mitochondrial disorders like Fibromyalgia, Chronic Fatigue Syndrome or premature aging. Top researchers in the field of neurodegenerative diseases suspect that illnesses like Parkinson's have a foundational basis in mitochondria malfunction. If your mitochondria are not doing their job it is impossible to be healthy.

What To Start Doing Right Now

Make sure you get the following supplements so your mitochondria can produce clean energy. Also you may want to consider

1. Magnesium Citrate: 450-600 mg a day

Magnesium is found in large concentrations inside your Mitochondria. It is needed for over 300 enzyme reactions that help produce energy. Magnesium is the single most important mineral for your health, although calcium seems to get all the attention. I have seen patients with restless leg syndrome completely cured after only one dose of magnesium citrate. I personally like the product, Natural Calm made by a company called Natural Vitality. I believe they are the best producer of magnesium citrate in the world. Start low in dose and build up to between 450-600 mg. a day. If you get loose stools cut back on the dose until your body adjusts. This is get way to reduce stress, relax the nervous system and produce effective Mitochondrial energy (ATP). This is also an essential cure for Restless Leg Syndrome because of the effect it has on relaxing the nervous system and muscle tissue.

2. Multi-B Complex: Daily

These vitamins provide the basic nutrition for the Mitochondria, a reason why some people feel more energized when they take B vitamins like B12. Your nerves have an insulation that grows around them known as a myelin sheath and the B vitamins are essential in the production of that material. This may not be a very exciting step, since everyone has heard about B vitamins but how many people are taking a B complex everyday, are you?

3. D3 (cholecalciferol not vitamin D2): 1000-2000 mg day

Cholecalciferol is really a hormone and not a vitamin. There is just so much research that indicates D3 deficiency can cause chronic muscle and joint pain,

9/10 people with chronic pain have a condition where they are deficient in D3.

I always run a serum 25-hydroxyvitamin D blood test to see where their levels are. Normal is considered 32-100 ng/ml but I am telling you that levels from 40-100 ng/ml are really much better. If you are in the low normal range start dosing. As a note, I live in Florida where there is beautiful sunshine everyday and I still see D3 deficiency.

4. Co Q-10: 100-200 mg a day

You want at least 200 mg a day and if you are currently suffering from an illness and you may need even more depending on your condition. It's now a proven fact that taking prescription Statin drugs which are taken for high cholesterol will reduce your body's Co-Q10 which can lead directly to heart disease. Does that make sense to you? Statins are a real problem but it is important to work with your doctor and not self manage them. In some cases they are needed but at the very least you can start taking Co-Q10, and consider dietary changes to eliminate the need for such dangerous drugs. I have good lab values but I take

Co-Q10 everyday because I know how important it is for my health.

Summary

To Activate Your Mitochondria

1. Magnesium Citrate: 450-600 mg a day
2. Multi-B Complex: Daily
3. D3 (cholecalciferol not vitamin D2): 1000-2000 mg day
4. Co Q-10: 100-200 mg a day

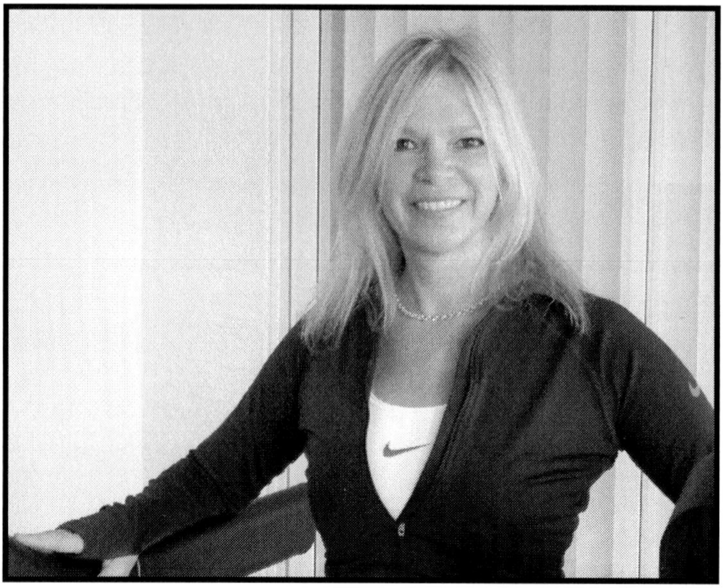

My wife Katherine is a perfect example of how regular exercise and proper diet can promote healthy hormonal production in women over 50 years of age. Although there is 8 years difference between us, I frequently have trouble keeping up with her.
I Love You Kathy.

Step Seven: Hormonal Regeneration

All you need in this life is a tremendous sex drive and a great ego. Brains don't mean a shit. -Captain Tony, Key West

Hormonal Testing

Mr. Cap Monroe lived in Southwest Florida and was 135 years old when he died. He swore that his longevity was because he drank a special tea made from Spanish Moss. This is a common moss that grows in the swamps, it hangs off the trees and is also known as Tillandsia Unsteadies. Since I live in Southwest Florida, I have started studying Spanish Moss and it turns out to contain mostly chlorophyll, minerals and B vitamins. So maybe Old Cap Monroe had discovered the fountain of youth after all. I am trying to manufacture a safe tea from the moss but honestly it is a nasty plant that houses insects and spiders. There are just better products available, not to mention the stuff tastes awful. Still I always think of old Cap Monroe whenever I go hiking down in the Everglades.

If there is one area of your health that you never want to guess at or self treat without proper knowledge it is hormones. Hormones are essentially chemicals that carry messages throughout your body. These chemicals have the power to pro-

duce miracles or they can destroy your body. So it is important to always, always test your hormone levels.
They are 3 main groups,

•Steroids which are made from cholesterol
•Lipids which are fats
•Amino Acids which make proteins and form brain chemicals called neurotransmitters.

Hormones have the power to produce miracles or they can destroy your body. So it is important to always test your hormone levels. This was difficult years ago but now it is simple and inexpensive. I personally do not care for urinary hormone testing because it is very inaccurate. The best way to test levels is with saliva testing and you can do this yourself, at home. One company that I have had great success using is ZRT Labs.

ZRT LABS 8605 SW Creekside Place, Beaverton, OR 97008
Phone: 1-866-600-1636 www.zrtlabs.com

They provide a big range of simple inexpensive tests that are non invasive and accurate. Both saliva and blood spot tests can be done in your own home without a doctor's prescription. The saliva test will check the following;

•Estradiol (E2)
•Estrone (E1)
•Estriol (E3)
•Progesterone (pg.)
•Testosterone (T)
•DHEA-S (Ds)
•Cortisol (C)

The blood spot test, is incredible and provides information on all these important markers;

•Estradiol (E2)
•Progesterone (Pg)
•Testosterone, total (T)
•DHEA-S
•Cortisol (C)
•Vitamin D: 25-OH Vitamin D2, 25-OH Vitamin D3, Total
•IGF-1 (Somatomedin C)
•Luteinizing Hormone (LH)
•Follicle-stimulating Hormone (FSH)
•Free Thyroxine (fT4)
•Free Triiodothyronine (fT3)
•Thyroid Stimulating Hormone (TSH)
•Thyroid Peroxidase Antibodies (TPO)
•Sex Hormone Binding Globulin (SHBG)
•Prostrate Specific Antigen (PSA)
•Fasting Insulin
•Total Cholesterol (CH)
•LDL Cholesterol
•HDL Cholesterol
•VLDL Cholesterol
•Triglycerides (TG)
•Hemoglobin A1c (HbA1c)
•High-Sensitivity C-Reactive Protein (hs-CRP)

You need to test these all these levels to really get a big picture of what is going on. Why wouldn't everybody get these tests? Knowing these levels will prevent many diseases before they get out of control. You can contact my clinic if you are interested in these or any other tests mentioned in this book.

What To Start Doing Right Now

Hormones are complicated and you should not start self treatment without first testing, however the following products are very safe regardless of your diagnosis and will benefit your overall hormone health without risk.

1. Progesterone Cream: Women 1/4 teaspoon, men 1/8 teaspoon 5 days a week.

Progesterone is safe, nontoxic and has many proven benefits for both men and women. It counters the dangerous effects of estrogen and balances estradiol and estrone. The prescribed oral progesterone is not the same thing. Real progesterone cannot be absorbed orally. Men need to understand how important progesterone is in preventing prostate cancer and premature aging. If you are a female over the age of 13 years old have your levels checked and get on some bioidentical transdermal cream and apply it according to your cycle. If you are post menopausal don't bother testing because you are no longer producing progesterone, just start applying the cream. Physicians have coined the term "estrogen dominance," to describe what happens when the normal ratio or balance of estrogen to progesterone is changed by excess estrogen or inadequate progesterone. Estrogen is a potent and potentially dangerous hormone when not balanced by adequate progesterone. Both women who have suffered from PMS and women who have suffered from menopausal symptoms, will recognize the hallmark symptoms of estrogen dominance:

•Weight gain
•Bloating
•Mood swings
•Irritability
•Tender breasts
•Headaches
•Fatigue
•Hypoglycemia
•Uterine fibroids
•Endometriosis
•Fibrocystic breasts
•Cancers- breast, ovary, endometrium (uterus) and prostrate

Men and women should take Progesterone as a transdermal cream. Taking Progesterone will counter the damaging effects of estrogen. Progesterone serves like a police officer in your hormonal system, protecting you against nasty things such as cancer. Progesterone trans dermal cream is available in most health food stores and on the internet without a prescription. Oral progesterone is not absorbed very well so rub this cream on areas of your body that have thin skin, like the insides of your wrists or upper chest. A good cream would be 500 mg of progesterone per ounce. Most progesterone creams come in 2 ounce containers so it should have at least 1000 mg.

Suggested Use: Postmenopausal women - apply 1/4 teaspoon to chest, stomach or abdomen any two weeks of the month. Premenopausal women - cycle from day 12 to 26 (day 1 is first day of period) by applying 1/2 teaspoon daily. Men - use 1/8 teaspoon five days of the week.

2. Melatonin: 1-5 mg 1/2 hour before bed,

Melatonin levels are directly related to how long you will live, how strong your immunity is, and how prone you are to getting cancer. Melatonin levels fall naturally as we age. This hormone regulates our internal clock. Mice given melatonin in their drinking water lived one-third longer than control mice. Imagine living to 100 rather than just 75 by taking melatonin. Get your levels checked at 3 am in the morning and use a saliva kit. Melatonin is quickly becoming one of the most powerful anti-aging hormones. The benefits of Melatonin can fill an entire book by itself. Here are some of its benefits according to the classic book,

The Melatonin Miracle, Nature's Age-Reversing, Disease Fighting, Sex-Enhancing Hormone by Walter Pierpaoli., M.D., PH.D., and William Regelson, M.D.

The book talks about using Melatonin to help with better sleep. This is common knowledge but it also explains melatonin's role in treating,

•AIDS
•Alzheimer's Disease
•Asthma
•Diabetes
•Down Syndrome
•Parkinson's Disease
•Poor Vision
•Sexual Dysfunction

The pineal gland is responsible for releasing melatonin and it is regulated by exposure to sunlight, increasing at night and dropping off during the day. It helps with many things but I believe the most important benefit is that it protects cellular DNA. It is now a well established fact that melatonin can slow down and even reverse aging. One of our newest threats to health are the electromagnetic fields that surround all our modern appliances. Cell phones, wireless computers, microwaves all produce energy fields that mess up our cellular DNA and cause cancer and sickness. These fields also deplete our body of melatonin. Supplementation is a good way to maintain healthy levels and counter the dangers of electromagnetic pollution.

3. Reduce Sugar Intake: The Anti-Hormone

Do not consume high sugar foods close to bedtime because these will stimulate insulin release and insulin suppresses growth hormone production. Most growth hormone production happens 1-2 hours after you go to sleep, so a high sugar meal before bed will destroy this process. Since GH supplementation is very expensive (thousands of dollars a month) and natural GH supplementation, in my opinion doesn't work, a better alternative is to work with the hormone you already have. Sugar is the enemy when it comes to all hormones, especially growth hormone. Remember white flour becomes sugar. So start by eliminating all the white trash products from your diet. Also sugar is sugar. You could be eating natural sugar cane, brown sugar, honey, maple syrup, agave, fructose, corn syrup, maltose or, xylitol but it is all sugar. Most commercial fruit juice on the market contains very little fruit juice and high amounts of high fructose corn syrup, so avoid it. Natural juice is not as bad because it has living enzymes that will help break down the sugars but it is still a high sugar food that needs to be limited. All sugar substitutes are dangerous and unhealthy.

Look at the kids today, they are mostly over weight, and 30% will develop diabetes. How did this happen? Sugar! We are the soda pop nation. I have more kids on diet programs than adults. The good news is just getting them off soda will make dramatic improvements to their health. If you are a parent throw out soda and save your child's life. Sucralose or Splenda is toxic. It states that it is made from sugar but that is not true. Sucralose is a synthetic halogenated, chemical soup full of chlorine which breaks down to dangerous unhealthy products in our body. Stevia is a plant extract and it is not safe either. The FDA has refused to approve Stevia as a sweetener until 2008 when they agreed to only approve the main alkaloid, Truvia, but not the whole extract. Stay away from Stevia, Aspartame, Nutrasweet and all sugar substitutes, they will harm you even more than sugar. You have to make a conscious effort to reduce and honestly eliminate your sugar intake if you have any chance of balancing your hormones without prescription drugs.

4. Have Sex! (This section contains adult material)

Got your attention? I cannot write a chapter on hormones without taking about sex. I get asked about sex a lot. For most people it is an embarrassing topic, not because sex is shameful but because sex is related to a primal purpose of reproduction and failure in this area really makes us feel disconnected from the Universe. The good news is that for 99% of the population suffering from sexual dysfunction it can be completely corrected.

So to avoid these uncomfortable discussions with patients I started giving them hand outs when they asked me for advice. You may not agree with this information but I can assure you that from a physiological perspective these self treatment techniques work. It's a fact that if you are not enjoying sex you will age faster and be more prone to disease. If you follow my 7 Steps To Innate Healing, you will resolve many sexual issues as your entire body starts to heal. There are a few bad habits like smoking and alcohol that need to be regulated because they reduce blood flow to the sex organs. Without proper blood flow orgasm will be difficult and eventually sexual desire will diminish and those important nerve receptors will start to desensitize. This creates chronic sexual dysfunction. Many prescription medications, like those taken for depression, blood pressure and heart disease also have a very negative effect on your sex life.

The basic ingredients to good sex is strong blood flow and a healthy neurological response. Walking is great to help with blood flow but if you are over weight it maybe hard on your joints. That is why I recommend you buy a recumbent bike. This allows you to sit down and peddle in the comfort of your own home. I like the inexpensive set of peddles you can buy at Wal-Mart, that way you can use your own chair and you can even place the peddles on a table top and peddle with your arms. This sort of exercise is used extensively in stroke rehab and with wheelchair patients but it works great for all of us. You can research upper body ergometers (UBE's) to get an idea of what I am describing. Start with 5 minutes twice a day and eventually work up to 30 minutes. Go slow. Alternate legs with arms, mix it up. Buy 2 units and do arms and legs at the same time, have some fun. This will really get your blood pumping through the body without placing stress on your back or joints. I have found adding oxygen to this procedure really increases effectiveness. You will need a doctors prescription to buy an oxygen concentrator but it should not be that difficult to get one. Breathing 3-5 lpm of oxygen while you are peddling is amazing. There is so much research on this that most athletes are currently doing some version of this. It is called exercise with oxygen therapy (EWOT). With this type of exercise you will be getting super oxygenated blood moving through your system. Your sex drive and performance will start to increase after only a few days of this type of training.

Now that we have you moving and are increasing blood flow throughout your body the next step is "neurological genital stimulation". That is my medical terminology (that I just made up) for telling you to get horny. I know this is uncomfortable material, believe me I know. I was told not to include this section of my book because it may offend some readers but this is important health information you may otherwise not get unless I tell you. Nerves will dies without stimulation so if you do not use this step you will not succeed. The cheapest way to stimulate growth of new neurological pathways to your genitals is with vibration. Go to Wal-Mart and buy a small back massager or hand vibrator. You do not need to go to a sex shop and buy an expensive penis shaped device (unless you want to) but you will need to vibrate the area, very gently and consistently. Maybe a few minutes once or twice a day. This will start the process of angiogenesis and new blood vessels and nerve pathways will start to form. Over about 14-28 days you will start getting more sensitivity in your pubic region, and more in touch, shall we say. Many times during this exercise you may find yourself reaching or close to reaching orgasm or not. There are no rules. Just continue to stimulate and over time things will start to happen for you. Where do you stimulate? Wherever it feels right, but be careful not to damage tissue with excessive friction. You only need very, very light stimulation. Men should stimulate between the scrotum and the rectum as well as gently along the sides of the penis. Women should stimulate the pubic bone and around the clitoris making sure not to injure the delicate tissues of the region. Some patients like using a water based lubrication. Experiment and decide for yourself. This is essential medical therapy, it is good for you and will help your overall level of health.

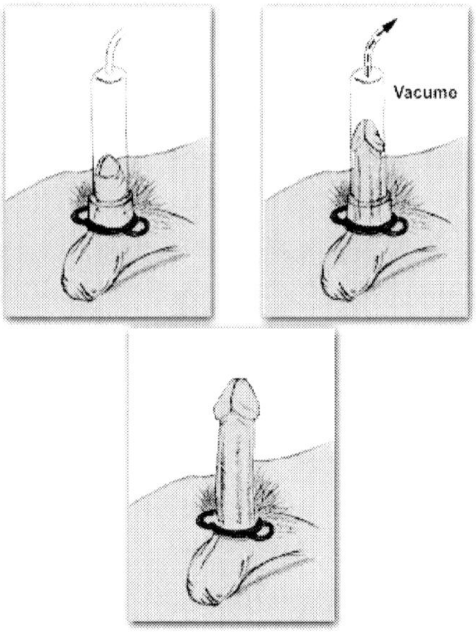

In most cases I will also recommend that men with erectile dysfunction use a vacuum constriction device (VCD). This is an external pump with a band on it that a man can use to get and maintain an erection. The VCD consists of an acrylic cylinder with a pump that may be attached directly to the end of the penis. A constriction ring or band is placed on the cylinder at the other end, which is applied to the body. The cylinder and pump are used to create a vacuum to help the penis become erect; the band or constriction ring is used to help maintain the erection. This is a medical treatment device and Medicare will pay for this equipment if you get a prescription. However you can buy the device yourself and it does not cost much at all. Regular use of the VCD will help stretch the blood vessels in the penis and allow easier blood flow. Regular use of the pump will train your penis and reactivate your sex life.

In theory, the gentle stretching should also stretch the suspension ligament that holds the penis, which will indirectly make your penis slightly longer.

Do I really need to say anything more about this? Seems to me like a no brainer, why not try it? You can get a prescription from your doctor or do like most patients and just buy it off the internet.

Sex is important, the more you have the better balanced your hormone levels will become. The important thing to remember here is that you must do these exercises even if you are currently having sex. This is your homework. Just having more sex is not the answer. Think of it like swinging a golf club. If your technique is bad then playing more golf will not make you swing better. The answer is you need to practice a correct swing. So practice. Practice makes perfect. Approach sex with a healthy, positive attitude (and have fun). Buy some books, talk to your doctor and pick up some relaxing music.

Extra Information: Testosterone is important for both men and women although men have about ten times more of it. It starts to decline as we get older and you really want to keep the levels that you had when you were in your 30's. You can use transdermal testosterone cream with is applied like the progesterone cream. Men can use about 3 mg daily and women 150 mcg. There is also good results with sublingual salts. You will need a medical prescription, see a physician trained in anti-aging medicine to get testosterone cream or sublingual salts.
The only non prescription product that seems to help with testosterone levels is Trebles. It can increase male and female libido. Trebles is an all natural herb that stimulates the Luteinizing Hormone, the hormone responsible for the body's testosterone production. There are quality issues with this product and you must be sure you are using the correct parts of the plant, the leaves and stems. The best source I have found is Tattva's Herbs. They have a product where they use 250 pounds of herb to make one pound of product, all organic super concentrated. But nothing is going to work like natural testosterone cream.

Now let's all take a cold shower and move on to the equally exciting world of neurotransmitters.

Neurotransmitters

Neurotransmitters are brain chemicals that help relay electrical messages from one nerve cell to another. They help regulate pain, reduce anxiety, promote happiness, initiate deep sleep and boost energy and mental clarity. They are very important in every healing mechanism your body uses and all neurotransmit-

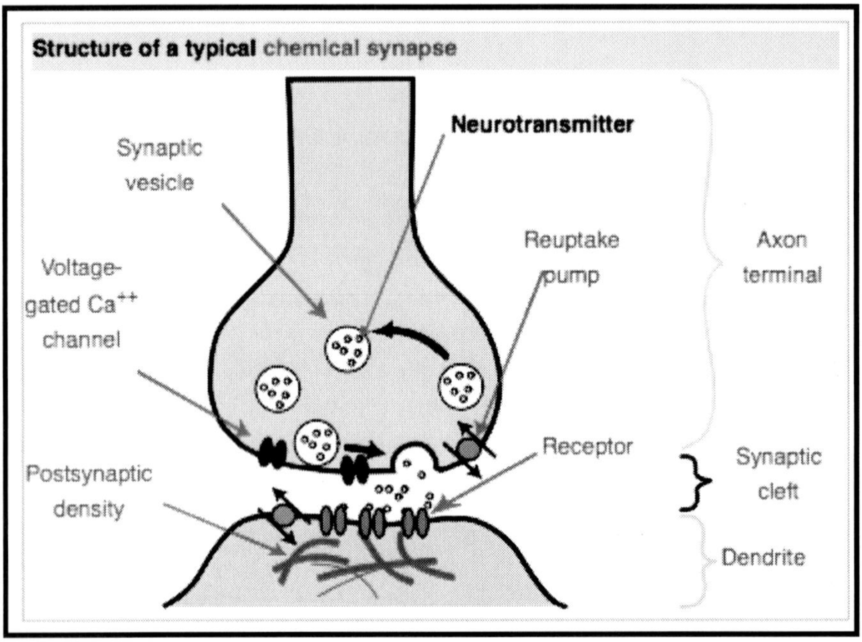

ters are made from amino acids. In the old days I got great results treating depression and many psychological disorders simply by having the patient drink a pint of beef broth every day. This was made from boiled down stew meat. The drink supplied all the amino acids the person needed to balance their neurotransmitters. Today, there are good supplements available and no need to drink the broth. Let's take a look at neurotransmitters and how they are related to your health.

DL-phenylalanine

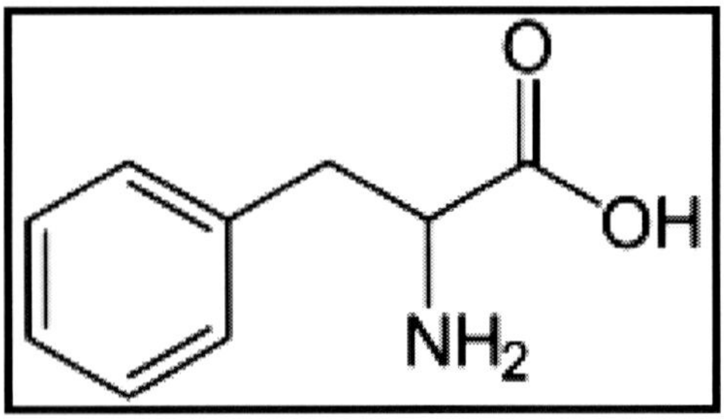

This is an essential amino acid and particularly beneficial in cases of chronic pain. If you are in pain and freaking out, just unable to handle it, this will really cut the edge for you and help you to feel better, almost right away. Phenylalanine is an essential amino acid (a building block for proteins in the body), meaning the body needs it for health but cannot make it. You have to get it from food. Phenylalanine is found in 3 forms:

- L-phenylalanine, the natural form found in proteins.
- D-phenylalanine (a mirror image of L-phenylalanine that is made in a laboratory).
- DL-phenylalanine, a combination of the 2 forms.

The body changes phenylalanine into tyrosine, another amino acid that's needed to make proteins, brain chemicals, including L-dopa, epinephrine, and norepinephrine, and thyroid hormones. Because norepinephrine affects mood, different forms of phenylalanine have been proposed to treat depression. Symptoms of phenylalanine deficiency include confusion, lack of energy, depression, decreased alertness, memory problems, and lack of appetite. On the other hand, a rare metabolic disorder called phenylketonuria (PKU) occurs in people who are missing an enzyme that the body needs to use phenylalanine. That causes high levels of phenylalanine to build up. If it is not treated before 3 weeks of age, PKU can cause severe, irreversible mental retardation. In the United States, newborns are tested for PKU during the first 48 - 72 hours of life. People with PKU must eat a diet that avoids phenylalanine and take tyrosine supplements to have optimum brain development and growth.

Dr. Arnold Fox, MD describes the antidepressant effects of DLPA in his book. First it increases the production of a brain stimulant called phenylethylamine. Furthermore, it inhibits the enzymes which break down the endorphin hormone. Endorphins regulate mood, so allowing them to hang around longer will make a person feel better. Finally, DLPA helps create norepinephrine, there have been multiple studies that show a strong connection between this chemical and depression. Most chronic pain sufferers will benefit from the addition of DLPA because most are depressed. I like putting my back pain patients on 750 mg of DLPA and have them take it with breakfast lunch and dinner, taken with meals. Dr. Fox's book is a great resource for DLPA therapy,

DLPA To End Chronic Pain and Depression Arnold Fox, M.D.

A study from the Brampton Brain Clinic suggests that DL-phenylalanine improves the action of other painkillers by increasing activity in the endogenous analgesia system. Disabled World notes that DL-phenylalanine has been shown to be particularly effective in patients who suffer from chronic pain due to conditions like arthritis. Another study led by H. Beckmann demonstrated that DL-phenylalanine worked as well as another common treatment in the reduction of depression symptoms, which has been linked in other studies to its role in the production of neurotransmitters. You can google these resources and investigate the research for yourself.

WARNING: You cannot use DLPA or L-tyrosine if you are taking MAO or tricyclic anti depressants.

L- tyrosine

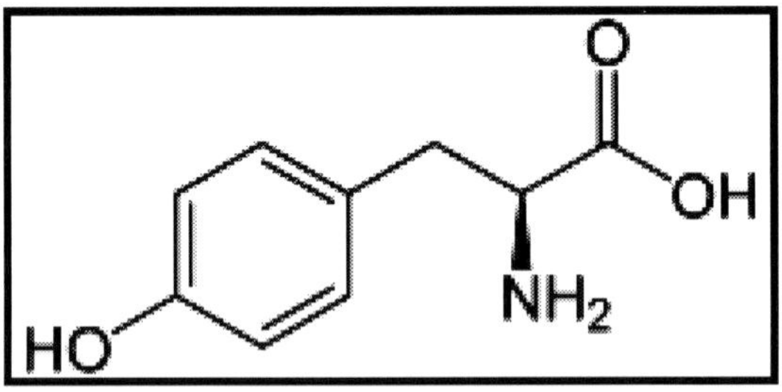

Improves memory, increases mental alertness, helps overcome depression and relieves obsessive compulsive disorder (OCD). There has been much research linking L-tyrosine deficiency to the increased craving of cocaine and alcohol. The best sources of L-tyrosine are meats, eggs and dairy products but it is hard to obtain the needed amounts in normal diets so supplementation is the desired way to get this product. Clinical studies show that L-tyrosine can control medication resistant depression when taken properly. My recommendation is 850 mg every morning and evening. Taking 25 mg of B6 will ensure you activate the L-tyrosine. I have a friend on the other coast who successfully treats addiction disorders with L-tyrosine and auriculotherapy.

WARNING: You cannot use DLPA or L-tyrosine if you are taking MAO or tricyclic anti depressants.

L- glutamine

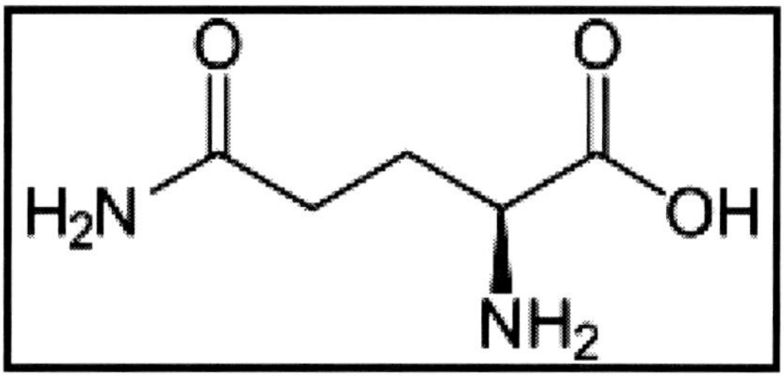

Is a precursor for GABA, the anti anxiety amino acid. New research demonstrates up to one third of the amino acids released during times of stress and anxiety is as glutamine. Under normal circumstances the body can make adequate amounts of the meal lasted but a prolonged stress, anxiety, panic, trauma or illness, the body cannot produce enough and requires glutamine supplementation. In patients who crave alcohol 3000 to 4000 milligrams of glutamine everyday can help. You can increase your IQ by taking between 500-1000 mg of Glutamine and I do use it with ADD and ADHD. Glutamine is converted to energy and is the brain's main fuel but it is also the main nutrient needed for intestinal repair. Whenever someone has a long history of NSAID abuse I always recommend glutamine to heal the gut, 1000-2000 mg divided up over 2 to 3 doses every day usually will produce dramatic results. Unfortunately, you just cannot get glutamine from food very good because cooking inactivates the amino acid, so your best source is supplementation, As with L-tyrosine B6 is a cofactor for activation.

5-hydroxytryptophan (5-HTP)

There has been much talk about this product. It is the precursor to serotonin in the brain which makes it super useful for overcoming many health problems. It is extracted from the Griffonia seed, which is a black flat circular seed that is found mainly

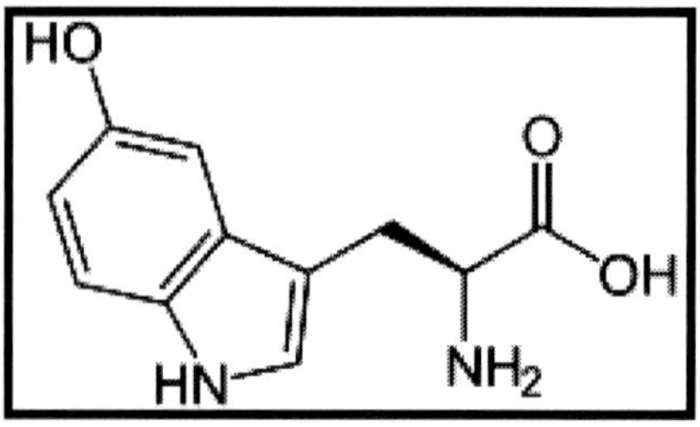

in Africa. Serotonin helps reduce anxiety, anger and aggression while it enhances sleep if you take it at bedtime.

WARNING: You cannot use 5-HTP if you are taking SSRI (selective serotonin repute inhibitors) or MAO inhibitors.

Clinically you should run a urine amino acid profile test to know how your body is handling these chemicals. Many individuals have "hidden" impairments in amino acid metabolism that are problematic and often go undiagnosed. These impairments may or may not be expressed as specific symptoms. They may silently increase susceptibility to a degenerative disease or they may be associated with, but not causative for, a disease. Because of the wealth of information provided, it is suggested that a complete amino acid analysis be performed whenever a thorough nutritional and metabolic workup is called for. Amino acid analysis provides fundamental information about nutrient adequacy: the quality and quantity of dietary protein, digestive disorders, and vitamin and mineral deficiencies (particularly folic acid, B_{12}, B_6 metabolism, zinc and magnesium). In addition amino acid analysis provides important diagnostic information about hepatic and renal function, availability of precursors of neurotransmitters, detoxification capacity, susceptibility to occlusive arterial disease (homocysteine), and many inherent disorders in amino acid metabolism.

In the clinic we use a company called Doctors Data,

Doctor's Data, Inc.
3755 Illinois Avenue
St. Charles, IL 60174-2420
U.S.A

I am including a copy of my clinical questions that I usually ask patients before neurotransmitter therapy. It directs us to the areas that need attention. I have found almost complete correlation between these questions and the amino profile.

Opioid

The following statements are often associated with patients who are in need of opioid neurotransmitter therapy.

•Your life seems incomplete.
•You feel shy with all but your closest friends.
•You have feelings of insecurity.
•You often feel unequal to others.
•When things go right, you sometimes feel undeserving.
•You feel something is missing in your life.
•You occasionally feel a low self-worth or self-esteem.
•You feel inadequate as a person.
•You frequently feel fear when there is nothing to fear.

Opioid neurotransmitters are contained in the hypothalamus gland. These neurotransmitters have two primary functions. First, opioids are released in small bursts when we feel a sense of urgency. Second when you exercise your body it releases extra opioids.

Recommendation: Start with DL-phenylalanine, take 1000 mg one - two times daily on an empty stomach. Keep increasing the dose up to 4000 mg twice a day. L-glutamine is also very effective and can increase the effectiveness of DL-phenylalanine. Take 500 mg one - two times daily on an empty stomach.

Some patients will experience rapid heartbeat, agitation or hyperactivity so do not take past three o'clock afternoon and remember with all neurotransmitter therapy always take the amino acids on an empty stomach.

GABA

GABA is an important neurotransmitter involved in regulating moods and mental clarity. Tranquilizers such as Xanax, Ativan and Klonopin are used to treat anxiety and panic disorders by increasing GABA. The following statements are often associated with patients who are in need of GABA neurotransmitter therapy.

•You often feel anxious for no reason.
•You sometimes feel free floating anxiety.
•You frequently feel edgy and it's difficult to relax.
•You often feel a knot in your stomach.
•Falling asleep is sometimes difficult.
•It's hard to turn your mind off and you want to relax.
•You experience feelings of panic for no reason.
•You often use alcohol or other sedatives to calm down.

Recommendation: GABA is made from the amino acid Glutamine. So we will start by taking a small dose, 500 to 1000 mg twice daily. Some individuals may need to take it 3 to 4 times a day, must be taken on an empty stomach. If you get a burning in the stomach or a flushing sensation substitute with L-theanine, 100-200 mg 2-3x a day on empty stomach and you should not have any problems.

As an interesting side note GABA does not normally cros sthe brain blood barrier, which means if you take GABA and you feel that it has an effect on you then there is a problem with your barrier. I will use this as a simple test on patients that I suspect a faulty brain blood barrier. If GABA is getting through chances are many other undesirables are also getting into the brain and causing problems.

Dopamine

Dopamine is that a neurotransmitter associated with the enjoyment of life: food, arts, nature, your family, friends, hobbies and other pleasures. Cocaine and chocolate's popularity stems from the fact that it causes very high levels of dopamine to be released in a sudden rush. The following statements are often associated with patients who are in need of Dopamine neurotransmitter therapy.

•You feel there is no real rewards in life.
•Unexplained lack of concern for others, even loved ones.
•You experienced decreased parental feelings.
•Life seems less colorful or flavorful.
•Things that used to be fun aren't any longer enjoyable.
•You have become a less spiritual or socially concerned person.

Recommendation: Brain cells that manufacture dopamine use the amino acid L-phenylalanine as a raw material. Start with 1000 mg of L-phenylalanine 1 to 2 times daily on an empty stomach. If you do not notice any benefits keep increasing the dose up to 4000 mg twice a day. Again you can also take L-glutamine, 500 mg one - two times daily on an empty stomach to increase the effectiveness. Alternative to L-phenylalanine is S-adenosyl-methionine (SAMe). Start with 200 mg on an empty stomach if you don't see improvement increase your dose by 200 mg each day up to 1200 mg until you do. SAMe can cause increase heart rate and blood pressure dry eyes and dry mouth. Do not take past 3 PM.

Norepinephrine

The neurotransmitter, norepinephrine causes feelings of arousal, energy and drive when released in the brain. Production of norepinephrine occurs in the hypothalamus and is a two-step process. The amino acid L-phenylalanine is first converted into tyrosine and then the tyrosine is converted into norepinephrine. The following statements are often associated with patients who are in need of norepinephrine neurotransmitter therapy.

•You suffer from a lack of energy.
•You often find it difficult to get going.

•You suffer from decreased drive.
•You also start projects and then don't finish them.
•You feel depressed.
•You occasionally feel paranoid.
•Your survival seems threatened.
•Your board great deal of the time.

Recommendation: Tyrosine can cause headaches, so start with 1000 mg of L-phenylalanine 1 to 2 times daily on an empty stomach. If you do not notice any benefits keep increasing the dose up to 4000 mg twice a day. As with most of the amino acids you can take L-glutamine, 500 mg one - two times daily on an empty stomach to increase the effectiveness. An alternative to L-phenylalanine is S-adenosyl-methionine (SAMe). Start with 200 mg on an empty stomach if you don't see improvement increase your dose by 200 mg each day up to 1200 mg until you do but do not take past 3 PM. as it can cause an increase heart rate and blood pressure.

Serotonin

Serotonin is a hypothalamus neurotransmitter necessary for sleep. The following statements are often associated with patients who are in need of serotonin neurotransmitter therapy.

•Hard for you to go to sleep.
•You can stay asleep.
•You often find yourself irritable.
•Your emotions lack rationality.
•You okay sure you experience unexplained tears.
•Noise bothers you more than it used to.
•You flareup and others more easily than he used to.
•You experience unprovoked anger.
•You feel depressed much of the time.
•You find you are more susceptible to pain.
•You prefer to be left alone.

Recommendation: 5-HTP, 100 to 200 mg at dinner and then again at bedtime should do the trick. Melatonin, mentioned earlier also is a precursor to serotonin.

There are several reasons why patients present with neurotransmitter problems,

•Low protein diets
•Magnesium deficiency
•Not enough essential fatty acids
•Stressful lifestyle
•Vitamin D
•Stimulants (caffeine, sugar, nicotine)
•Adrenal fatigue
•Thyroid function

Adrenal Glands

Your body has a system designed to deal with stress, it is called the adrenal system. The hormones secreted by your adrenals influence every major physiological process in the body. How you heal, how fast you age and whether you get sick are all directly related to healthy adrenal glands.

Many times I'm forced to give patients a prognosis on whether a specific treatment program is going to work. Of course this is totally impossible and I really hate to place some sort of percentage on a patients chance of getting better. I always tell them, they have every reason to expect a positive outcome because under ideal circumstances the body will heal itself. It is our job to provide a healthy environment and then get out of the way so innate can do it's thing. Still, if the adrenal system is not functioning correctly the body will have difficulty dealing with the healing process and when you think about this it makes perfect sense. Someone who is spending all of their energy on dealing with stress will have very little left over for healing.

So about five years ago I started testing the adrenals on every patient before I accepted them into care. The test is very simple, a small amount of urine is taken and is mixed with silver nitrate, than drop by drop potassium chromate is mixed into the solution. The mixture will eventually turn orange at which point you can determine the status of the adrenal glands. A system that is hyperactive is just as detrimental as one that is hypoactive. I recorded these results and found a direct correlation between adrenal health and recovery. Today just about every patient I see takes an adrenal supplement while they are receiving therapy in my office and it allows us to be much more aggressive in the approach. With adrenal support they just get better faster and are less sore after treatment.

One way you can assess the status of your adrenal system at home is by simply taking your blood pressure while you're lying down and then standing up and taking it again. What we are most interested in here is the systolic blood pressure. This is the first number or the high number in your blood pressure reading. So in a normal blood pressure of 120/80 the systolic number is the 120. Your systolic pressure should go up about 10 points or more when you stand up and walk around for a few seconds. If your systolic pressure stays the same, goes down or only goes up a few points you most likely have a problem with your adrenal glands. This is a simple test and although not as accurate as the urine test it is a good way to do a quick home assessment. What you don't have a blood pressure cuff? Go buy one today, blood pressure is just one of those indicators you need to keep a close eye on if you are interested in staying healthy.

If you are experiencing adrenal fatigue the first solution is get more sleep. That's simple enough, rest more often and for longer periods of time. If your blood pressure tends to run low you can add more salt and water to your diet. Obviously do not start increasing salt if you have congestive heart failure or high blood pressure but salt is a natural antihistamine and helps reduce pain and inflammation, so it is not always a bad thing. Although there are fancy supplements on the market for the adrenals I like plain and simple vitamin C.

Start with 1000 mg and increase until you have loose stools and then decrease by 500 mg until your bowels normalize.

Adrenal gland supplementation is complex and you cannot self administer. If you continue to have adrenal problems make an appointment and see a doctor who is trained in functional medicine. I use glandular extracts and DHEA all the time with great results but they can be dangerous so it is best to not gamble with your health. Besides, I am only a phone call away.

Thyroid Gland

People are going crazy over thyroid problems. Here in South West Florida I see newspaper ads every week focused on thyroid disease. The ads list many of the related symptoms. Even my wife Katherine wanted to get tested after seeing these ads and frankly it's not a bad idea because thyroid disease is on the rise. Most people never think about testing their thyroid levels or even worse they get the thyroid tested but only check TSH. That's no good. If you have been placed on replacement thyroid hormones only based on a TSH test, please get more testing. The problem with TSH is that it will vary from day to day making it unreliable. You need to get your free T3 and free T4 tested, this is the key. Also your thyroid maybe the victim of an autoimmune attack that is spiking levels, so you must really be careful here.

Another problem with thyroid testing is the "normal ranges". Your doctor will usually look at your tests and if they are in range he will assume everything is fine but I don't agree with this. Lets say you are a 1.7 on a 1.5 to 2.5 scale (average of 2.0) for T3, you may be considered in range but really you are low. If this is your level then you should consider raising it with bioidentical triiodothyronine. If you are a 10 on a 7 to 25 scale (average of 16) for T4 you are not normal. Yes, you are in range but you are low. Use bioidentical L-thyroxine and raise your T4 level. A common mistake people make is using Armour pig thyroid but because it contains both T3 and T4 it is counterproductive.

Here are the symptoms of an under active thyroid
•Fatigue
•Weight gain
•Excessive appetite
•Depression
•A general tired feeling
•Irritability
•Feeling cold
•Thinning hair
•Difficulty in concentration
•Infertility
•High blood fats

If you have a low, out of range, free T3 level, you can consider a basic dose of 25 mcg of Synodal (triiodothyronine) as a starting point. If you find you have a low, out of range, free T4 level, you can consider a basic dose of 100 mcg of Levelly (L-thyroxine) as a starting point. It is always a 4 to 1 ratio of T4 to T3 in mammals. Everyone is different, and only blood monitoring over time will tell you which dose you personally need. Again as I always tell patients, hormones are the key to everything but do not self treat without knowledge. Get tested, find a knowledgable physician and continue with caution. If you mess around with these stuff without knowing what you are doing you will destroy your health.

Symptoms of overactive thyroid include,
•High pulse
•High blood pressure
•Osteoporosis
•Vision problems
•Restlessness
•A feeling of being nervous
•Bulging eyes (in extreme cases)

Overactive thyroid is much harder to treat. Do not allow some undereducated medical doctor to poison (using methimazone), destroy (with radioactive iodine), or remove your thyroid gland (with surgery) to slow down hormone production. Correct diet, healthy lifestyle, proven supplements, and balancing your other hormones will help normalize your levels. All your hormones work together as a team so balance them all, start anywhere, just do it.

Many people believe that Synthroid, which is simply T4, and Cytomel, which is simply T3, are somehow not natural. Nonsense. Both of these are completely bioidentical. Again get a good physician who can prescribe these medications and make sure you monitor yourself after 90 days to see if you are taking the correct dose. I tell patients to monitor yearly after that. Again, please remember that all your basic hormones should be balanced for your thyroid to operate well. Diet and lifestyle will do wonders for your thyroid gland.

Warning: The information given here is only for educational purposes. Get tested and get under medical observation. Work with your doctor and together solve your thyroid condition. In my practice I always work with the patient's endocrinologist when suggesting hormonal therapy.

Summary

Know Your Hormone Levels:

1. Saliva Hormone Panel Test (ZRT Labs)
2. Neurotransmitter Urine Evaluation (Doctor's Data)
3. Adrenal Fatigue Panel
4. Thyroid Panel

Hormone Balancers:

1. Progesterone Cream: 1/8- 1/4 teaspoon 5 days a week.
2. Melatonin: 1-5 mg 1/2 hour before bed
3. Get Off Sugar.
4. Have Sex!
5. Take Specific Neurotransmitter Stimulators
6. Heal The Adrenals
7. Balance The Thyroid

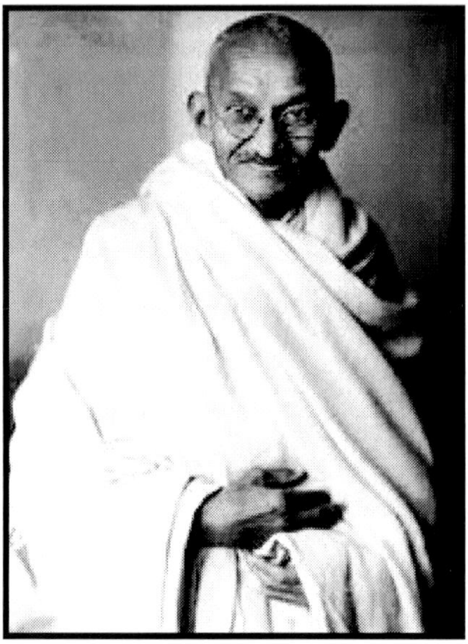

When I despair, I remember that all through history the ways of truth and love have always won. There have been tyrants, and murderers, and for a time they can seem invincible, but in the end they always fall. Think of it--always.

-Mahatma Gandhi

Conclusion

Science cannot solve the ultimate mystery of nature. And that is because, in the last analysis, we ourselves are... part of the mystery that we are trying to solve. -Max Planck, Physicist

This is an ironic title for the last chapter in this book because there is no conclusion to healing yourself, the process is forever ongoing. Health cannot be neatly packaged in a few hundred pages. Remember generality will provide more powerful results than specialization. It is impossible to isolate hormone concerns from digestion or mitochondria disorders from autoimmune disease. This is the theme of my book, everything must be observed and treated together in a holistic (treat the whole) format. Many times when something seems to not respond, despite great effort it is a good idea to leave it, temporarily perhaps and review another system. For example, if you are unable to improve your adrenals maybe you just need to help your liver detoxify better. Perhaps nociceptor pain signals that are constantly being stimulated from a herniated lumbar disc needs to be addressed. The body is a closed circuit so everything works together, like a group of singers, all different, coming together to produce a beautiful song that is in tune. Working on the individual parts always improves the whole. The Universe has granted us the ability to heal ourselves. A human body operating correctly does not get sick. There are many details in this book, don't get overwhelmed and what is more important, do not become obsessed about things, like your diet. Do the best you can. Not everyone is designed to be 100 pounds or live 100 years. We must accept who we are and enjoy the precious gift we have been given. My dad would always say to me,

You cannot push a piece of string.

Please accept yourself. We are designed individually to have slightly different experiences while on this planet. This is the freedom, and the beauty of life but also it's curse. The time we are alive is short and human life is so incredibly precious, do not waste your time chasing other peoples ideals. Follow your own. I am convinced that every human being is important and useful. Our purpose, is to fulfill our genetic expression, whatever that maybe. Work with whatever God has granted you, allow your body the opportunity to live at it's maximum potential. Please open your eyes and see for the first time your importance in the cosmic soup.

Love is what's left when you let go of everything that you don't need.

These are words to live by. I wish you sincere happiness and connection to the Universe through innate intelligence.

-Stephen

The Bonus Lecture: Herbs

Whatever you can do, or dream you can do, begin it. Boldness has genius, power, and magic in it.
-Johann Wolfgang von Goethe

Herbs are powerful medicine and should be considered with the same respect as prescription drugs. Do not take then without proper, professional guidance. Just like you would not take someone's heart medicine you should not take herbs without knowledge. They have the power to heal but can also make you very sick if misused. Herbs are not part of our normal physiology like vitamins and minerals, so they are not intended to be taken forever. Usually I like to alternate herbs in a 6 month cycle depending on what is being used. In the next few pages I am giving you my clinical notes on some herbs that I have found to be very effective, meaning they do what they are supposed to do. It seems funny to say that but most products on the market do nothing or will make patients sick. Also you need to get these herbs from a good source. I import herbs directly from organic farms in India. If you are buying them on your own and not from a physician you should shop around and do some research. Below is a transcription of a lecture I recently gave where I discussed several of my favorite herbs that produce stellar results. Dosages will depend on the severity of the condition and history.

The Lecture

There are two herbs, **Albizia** and **Skullcap**, which stabilize mast cells and reduce the amount of histamine released. They are herbal antihistamines. Anytime a patient presents with allergies, no matter what the cause these herbs can have a profound effect. Symptoms such as itchy eyes and runny noses or allergic skin conditions related to eczema, dermatitis and psoriasis can be helped by these herbs. Many times I will also add Echinacea.

Whatever I need a very strong immune modulator I will prescribe **Echinacea**. It works great with skin disorders such as psoriasis, acne, eczema or for any short-term treatment of infectious conditions such as influenza, colds, cystitis, shingles particularly those of a chronic or recur in nature. Quality is extremely important when dealing with echinacea because in human trials it is the alkylamides of the Echinacea that was the only chemical found in human plasma samples. It's important to use echinacea at the first signs of infection. This usually stops the infection in its tracks. It is important to remember that besides being an immune enhancer Echinacea is also an immune modulator and has much value in treating many autoimmune conditions. Echinacea has anti-inflammatory properties which make it ideal for incorporating into many different types of protocols. I see great improvements and skin conditions using echinacea. It is definitely one of my top herbs that I use everyday.

When it comes to treating the eye, **Bilberry** is the herb. It improves visual acuity which in turn improves sight. It's beneficial to any condition that is associated with impaired microcirculation. I use it regularly for macular degeneration but also see incredible results in patients with diabetic retinopathy. Combined with ginkgo you get very powerful results.

Inflammation is a common player in just about every disease process. Clinically I can relieve pain and inflammation associated with arthritis, endometriosis, IBS, Crohn's disease, ulcerative colitis and psoriasis, with a combination of **Boswellia**, **Turmeric** and **Ginger**. These inhibit inflammatory leukotrienes which reduces cellular inflammation. This stuff also works good for the treatment of asthma, were leukotrienes are a major cause inflammation. Because inflammation is such a common factor, I prescribed some combination of these herbs with almost every patient.

Cats Claw is good for anyone suffering from fungal infections I especially like using it in cases where the patient is over run with Candida. It has a valuable role to play as an adjunct to therapy for patients with cancer and leukemia and it's beneficial to counter the immunosuppressive effects of conventional cancer treatment. In those cases I like to combine that with **Essay**.

My number one herb for premenstrual syndrome would be **Chaste Tree.** In my clinical practice it works 100% of the time. It also has benefit for infertility in both men and women is a major herb for the treatment of acne.

Recently, there's been talk about the benefits of essential fatty acids. Unfortunately, most of the products on the market are tainted and end up producing the opposite effect from which they were intended. In my opinion the oil that has the most clinical data supporting its efficiency is **Evening Primrose Oil**. EPO is a registered drug in England for treating diabetic neuropathy and delivers a good herbal source of gamma linolenic acid. Besides taking a capsule you can also apply GPO transdermally. This is a good method of delivery specially for children where I'll have the mother simply cut the top of the capsule and rub the oil on the skin so it can be absorbed into the bloodstream, most children don't like taking capsules.

Feverfew. Well, for me this is the treatment for migraine headaches. For a while it was very popular but then it seemed to die off because many people were claiming it didn't produce a very strong therapeutic benefit. The problem with feverfew is that you can't take a couple of tablets for a week and expected to have any effect on your migraines; you really need 3 to 6 months of continuous use for it to have on effect on migraines. As you're taking it, you will notice that drugs like aspirin or acetaminophen will work more effectively so you won't need to take as much of those medicines while you're waiting for the feverfew to take over. Typically in my clinic I will combine Feverfew with White Willow Bark to help with migraine headaches and then usually some other herbs depending on what the root cause of the migraine is, many times I'll add Chaste Tree if there are hormonal imbalances.

I use medicinal mushrooms, especially in cases where the immune system is compromised, such as chemotherapy patients, post viral symptoms, HIV infection or autoimmune diseases. To the most popular would be the **Shiitake** and the **Ganoderma**. Of course, echinacea usually plays a part in those protocols as well.

Any time I need to lower blood lipid levels such as in the treatment or prevention of artery disease, hypertension or a situation where I just need to improve peripheral circulation like diabetic neuropathy, I like using **Garlic** as an acid resistant tablet. Usually I will see clinical results in as little as four weeks.

One of my personal favorite herbs is **Ginkgo**. Many studies that show it improves short-term memory mental alertness cognitive function and circulation to the brain hard eyes ears and legs. It's a good herb for people suffering from dementia or early onset of Alzheimer's disease. I will usually prescribed to go in cases of tinnitus and vertigo. It's a great product but you need to be aware that there are many quality issues associated with ginkgo, so it's very important to get high quality herb. The effects of ginkgo on concentration is almost immediate and therefore can be taken right before performing any cognitive function for improved results. If I am giving a lecture, I will normally take 3 or 4 Ginkgo tablets before the presentation and it gives me the edge.

Problems that involve the mucous membranes, such as upper respiratory problems, intestinal dysbiosis or ENT disorders usually respond well to **Golden Seal**. When a mucus is green I always think to use golden seal.

Angiogenesis is the process by where the body grows new blood vessels and it's really essential in most healing. Any herb that increases blood flow in the body will usually aid in healing process and one herb that I especially like for tissue healing is **Goto Kola**. I will always use this to promote healing and to prevent adhesions from forming after surgery or tissue injury. It's good for damaged discs and especially good for diabetic neuropathy patients who are suffering with ulcers and reduced circulation. This herb is so powerful and necessary that I prescribe it to just about every patient.

Hawthorne is an herb that the Germans call "The nurse of the elderly heart". It has a number of actions that benefit the heart. It lowers the oxygen requirements of the heart muscle and promotes re-vascularization of the heart. Most of the time I prescribed along with ginkgo for stellar results. It also lowers blood pressure but usually requires a month or two to take effect.

Gastritis, ulcers, acid reflux, heartburn, and indigestion are usually lifestyle driven conditions. **Licorice Root** is very effective in healing the gastric mucosa but it is contraindicated in patients with hypertension or edema which usually coexists in many patients with gastric inflammation. So my clinic, I will use licorice root that has been deglycyrrhizinized to avoid any adverse reaction.

In the ancient world there was a saying, all roads lead to Rome. In healthcare all roads lead the liver. The joke among doctors is when you don't know what to do next or you never knew what to do in the first place, treat the liver. I like **Milk Thistle** seed for the protective support it gives the liver but milk thistle seed has very little influence on detoxification. For that I like to use rosemary leaf. Anytime I get a case of toxin overload poor liver function, over indulgence in alcohol or rich fatty foods I always prescribe these herbs. Also any patients who frequently take prescription medication particularly acetaminophen will need this type of support.

Two plants I like to combine are **Ginseng** and **Rhodiola**. This is my basic vitality formulation. I also use it as part of my male infertility program. It is excellent for improving performance and reducing recovery time when exercising.

White Willow Bark is my number one prescription for reducing pain. It's been proven in many clinical trials to be effective and usually produces results within 48 hours. I like to combine it with **Boswellia** to knock out the inflammation that usually accompanies pain syndromes.

Most people already know that **St. John's Wort** is an effective antidepressant but very few people know it also is a very strong antiviral. I prescribe it frequently in combination with immune enhancing herbs for viral infections such as herpes, Epstein-Barr virus and other envelope viral infections. It will not work on non-enveloped viruses like human papaloma virus, which causes warts. Most of the hepatitis viruses are envelope the exception of hepatitis A which is non-envelope.

Unfortunately male and female fertility and libido dysfunction are on the rise in America, likely due to a combination of toxin exposure and stressful lifestyle. **Trebles** is a fantastic herb but it has many quality issues. For results you need to use the right part of the plant, the leaves and stems, that were used in clinical trials. Although Trebles grows all over the world the plants grown in Central Europe contains the most important constituent, protodioscin. This extract is the secret ingredient to many highly respected medical fertility experts high success rates.

Valerian is excellent for insomnia or people that have difficulty falling to sleep. Irritability, restlessness, anxiety and nervous tension respond well to Valerian.

There's much talk these days about antioxidants and anti-aging in the media. There is a current theory known as the free radical theory of disease that suggests just about all disease is the result of free radical buildup in the body. It has been my own experience that free radicals certainly play a major role in aging and degeneration. I suggest all my patients, without exception, take a good combination of antioxidant herbs on a regular basis. Complex herbal antioxidants are more beneficial and safer than single antioxidants. My experience has been a combination of **Green Tea, Turmeric, Grape Seed Extract and Rosemary Extract** produces the strongest response.

I work with many women and **Wild Yam** is one of the mainstays. I find it absolutely fantastic for the treatment of menopausal symptoms. Patients rave about the results. Is very effective in reducing many of the common symptoms of menopause including hot flashes, night sweats, insomnia, mood changes, fatigue, reduce mental function and reduce physical endurance.

Ten years ago I lectured about adrenal fatigue and was met with resistance from the medical community. Today, adrenal fatigue is all over the media and it is an accepted diagnosis. A simple test that many people can do on their own involves taking blood pressure when you're lying down and then retaking the pressure once you stand up. The first number or the high number (the systolic pressure) should increase as you move from a reclined position to a standing position. If it stays the same or decreases there's a strong chance that your adrenal system is not keeping up. In the clinic we also do a test with silver nitrate known as Konsberg's test. It uses 10 drops of urine from the patient and can tell if they are suffering from adrenal fatigue or adrenal stress, a very useful, inexpensive test. To treat I like the combination of **Korean Ginseng** and **Ashwaganda** and sometimes I add Licorice and Skullcap to cover all the bases. This is excellent for type A personalities and those that are wound up, yet run down. It boosts energy, stamina and releases nervous tension. I also notice that it will improve appetite in children.

It's hard to imagine but hygiene is still a big problem for some people. There many reasons for this including our relationships with domestic animals and the close living arrangements found in many of our big cities. Cleanliness is a much bigger problem than people understand and usually leads to harmful parasites and worms. In those cases where we see infestation, **Wormwood** is it herb that takes effect almost immediately. Usually it will get rid of all symptoms within three days. This is a more mainstream problem than people think.

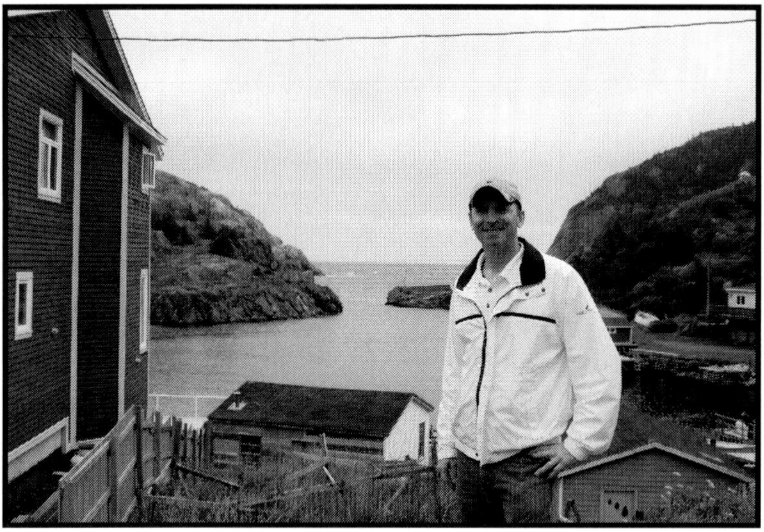

Quidi Vidi fishing village (pronounced Kiddy Viddy) is just a few minutes walk from where I was born in St. John's. I visited recently while attending the funeral of my grandfather Frank Stokes. Today's weather was the same as always, rain drizzly and fog. -Dr. Stokes

The Author

Personal Life

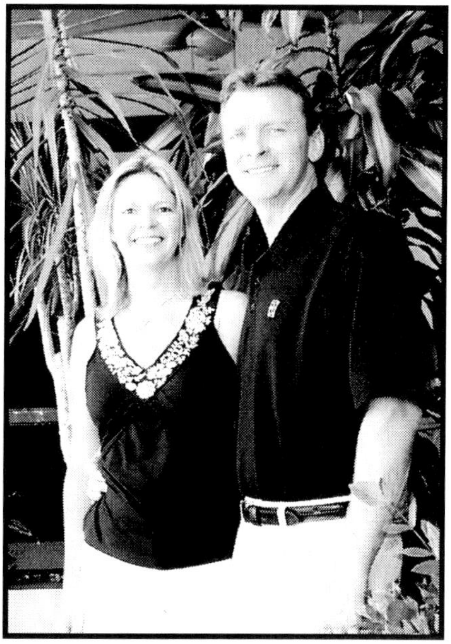

During the last decade I have operated many successful clinics, all with the help of my wife Katherine. Together we have guided thousands of patients towards self healing. This continues to be our life purpose. I believe in the human potential to do good things. Although some of us get lost, we must remain faithful in the basic belief that people are good. With proper focus there is nothing we cannot achieve. In my third book, I am writing extensively on the subject of miracles and the ability to achieve supernatural consciousness. For most of us we are never aware that there is an invisible world existing in synchronicity with our perceived reality. By using simple tools like the power of intent, we can access this other reality and change anything in our lives. This information will challenge what you believe is possible and alter the way you think about your purpose on this planet. Stay tuned, it will be a wild ride down the rabbit hole.

I enjoy many pastimes and hobbies but reading is my favorite. Naturally I collect books and have a very good library of ancient, esoteric writings. In my quest for hidden knowledge I participate in several fraternal brotherhoods. I am a Freemason, Royal Arch Mason and Companion of Cryptic Masonry. I am a Noble of the Mystic Shrine, member of the Knights of Malta, Order of the Red Cross and have been knighted under the jurisdiction of the Grand Commandery of the Knights Templar of Florida (commandery #32). Through these organizations I actively support the Shriner Children's Hospital Program and I am a life time sponsor of the Knights Templar Eye Foundation, Inc.

You can usually find me meditating before sunrise and staying fit with routine fasting and a special set of exercises that I was taught while studying the works of the late Dr. Robert Fulford. I highly recommend everyone read, The Philosophical Physician and learn more about this unique healer.

I am formally trained in several martial arts (Wing Chun, Jeet Kune Do, Kali, Escrima, Kendo and Judo), but no longer practice the hard path. Mistakenly, I have raised the Kundalini and was bitten by the snake. This was a very unpleasant experience from which I am still recovering. Playing with energy is dangerous and if you decide on exploring get training to avoid getting burned.

I have a step son, Michael, who is attending St. Louis University. I also have a sister, Raylene, who practices law in St. John's, Newfoundland (Canada). Her husband Mark runs McCarthy's Party, a high energy internationally praised tour company. I have two children by my first marriage, Micheal and Gabrielle, who I miss terribly.

Katherine and myself support ACT, Abuse Counseling and Treatment, Inc. which is a private agency committed to serve victims of domestic violence, sexual assault and human trafficking. We believe in helping others through service and are open to those in need. Many times I find myself falling into the trap of empathy. This is the greatest problem with healers. It is important to care and help but never cross your own energy with the patient's otherwise they will make you sick. These energy vampires really exist, I see them everyday.

As a physician, I have witnessed many miracles in the lives of my patients and myself. Over the years I have accepted my role as a facilitator and understand that all healing comes from The Great Architect,

I Am What I Am
J*h*v*h

Vi veri universum virus vici

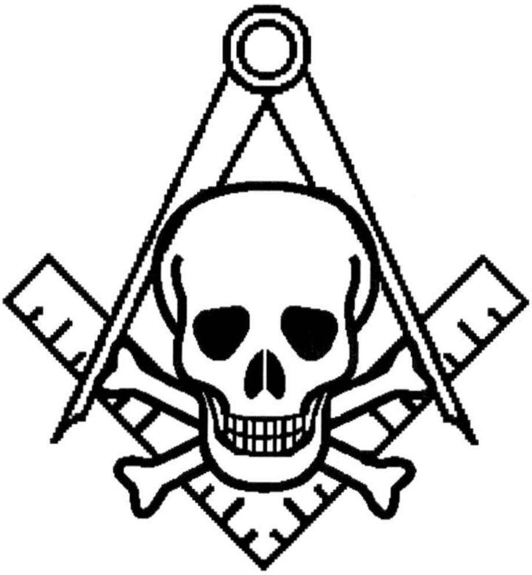

So Mote It Be